AMERICAN JOURNAL of PUBLIC HEALTH
OCTOBER 2023
Issue 10

AJPH

A PUBLICATION OF THE
AMERICAN PUBLIC HEALTH ASSOCIATION

FINDING COMMON GROUND FOR PUBLIC HEALTH ACTION

Building Common Ground, p. 1093
The Proof by COVID-19, p. 1036
Practical Principles, p. 1106
Information Quality, p. 1096
Crosscurrents Dialogue Model, p. 1099
Generation Z, p. 1114
Beyond “Surveillance,” p. 1102

Also in this issue:

MENTAL HEALTH
Among US Youths, p. 1116

RISK FOR MPOX
Stigmatizing Policies, p. 1120

INDIGENOUS PEOPLE
Cultural Safety in Public Health, p. 1059

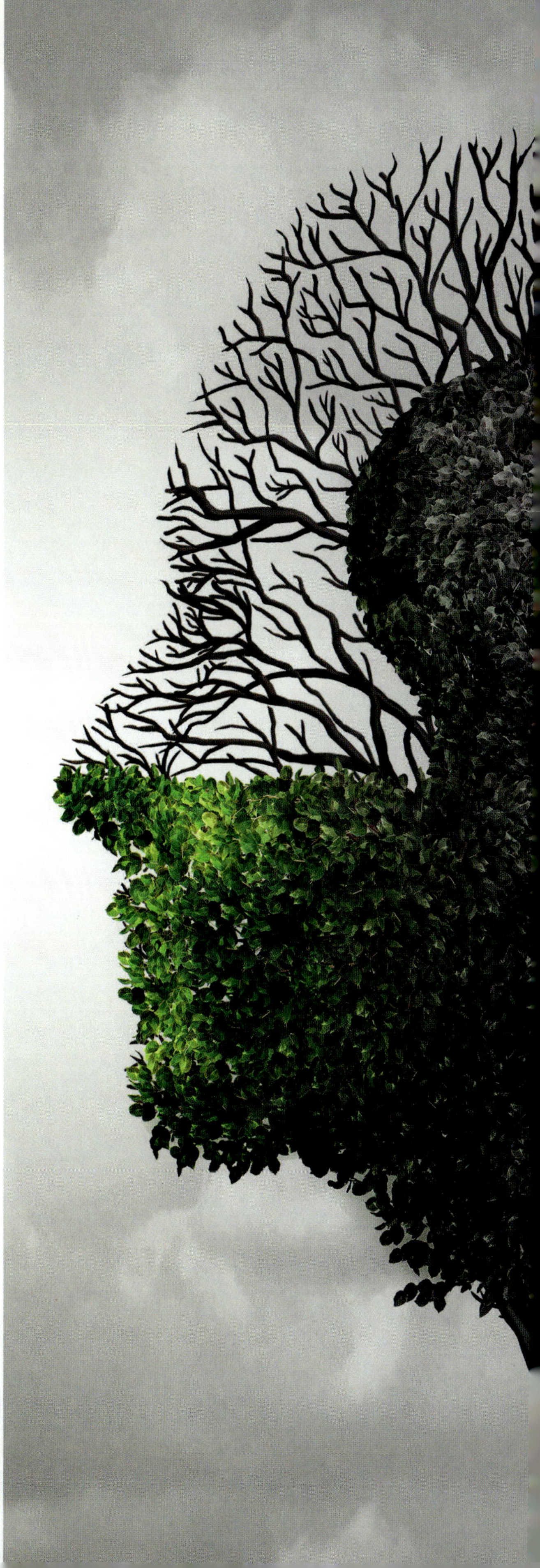

When It Comes To Health, Never Compromise. Choose Quality Rubber Medical Devices.

Good health is not something money can buy. However, choosing high-quality, reliable medical devices certainly is. **Made in Malaysia** quality rubber medical devices are produced to meet stringent international standards and are exported worldwide. Malaysian manufacturers have esteemed reputations, using modern manufacturing facilities to produce a wide range of quality rubber medical devices such as examination gloves, surgical gloves, condoms, foley catheters, dental dams, breathing bags, and medical tubing at competitive prices. When it comes to rubber, **No One Knows Rubber Like Malaysia Does.**

Reach Malaysian manufacturers via Marketplace at **www.myrubbercouncil.com**

NO ONE KNOWS RUBBER LIKE MALAYSIA DOES

Conform to International Standards	World's No. 1 in Natural Rubber Gloves & Nitrile Gloves	Made in Malaysia Quality Rubber Products	Wide Range of Rubber Medical Devices

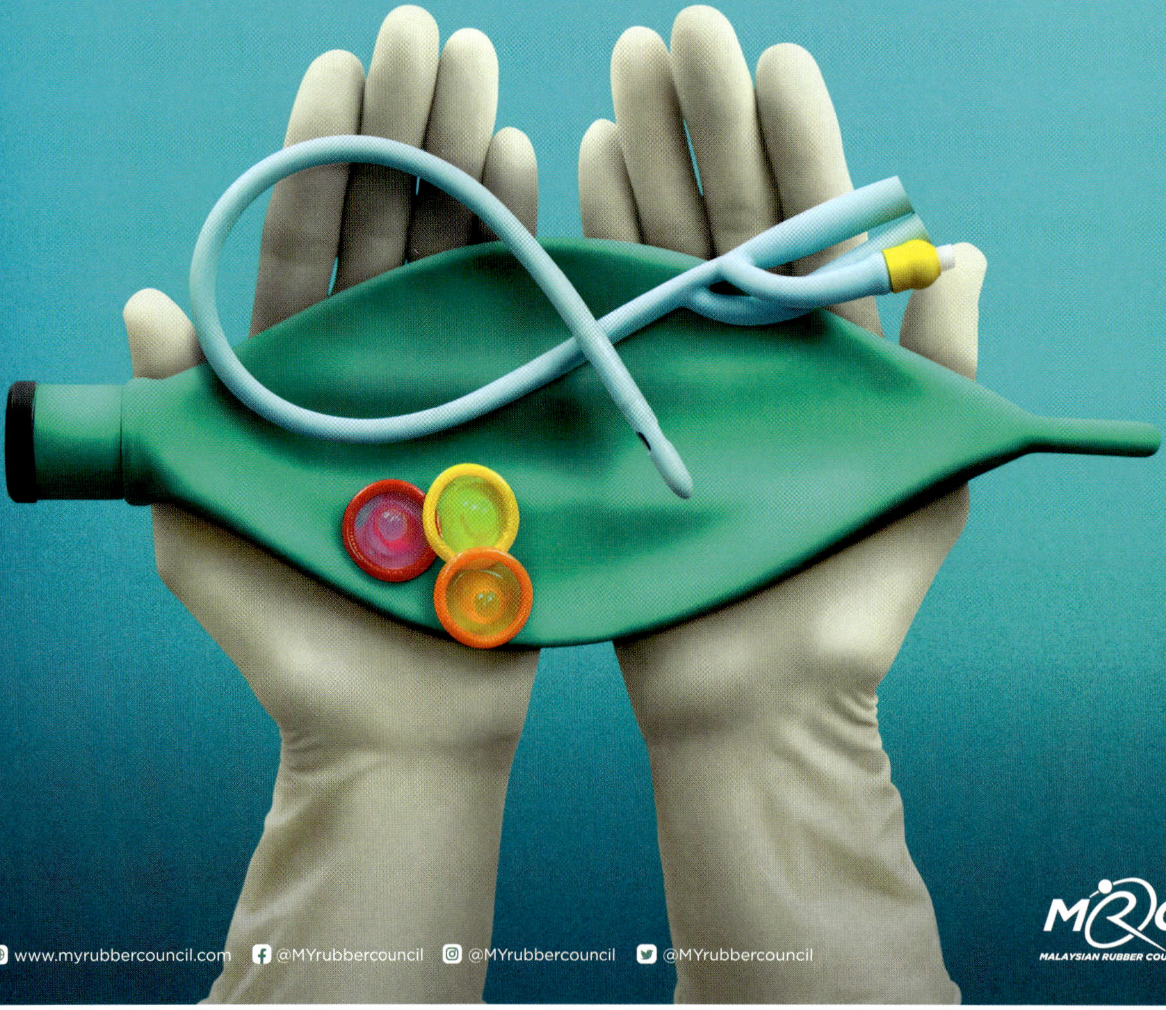

www.myrubbercouncil.com @MYrubbercouncil @MYrubbercouncil @MYrubbercouncil

MRC MALAYSIAN RUBBER COUNCIL

APHA
AMERICAN PUBLIC HEALTH ASSOCIATION
For science. For action. For health.

AJPH®, published monthly, is the official Journal of the American Public Health Association®, 800 I St NW, Washington, DC 20001-3710; (202) 777- APHA; TDD (202) 777-2500. APHA is a nongovernmental professional society founded in 1872, representing all disciplines and specialties in public health.

The *American Journal of Public Health*® (*AJPH*) (print ISSN: 0090-0036; electronic ISSN: 1541- 0048), first published in 1911, is the official journal of the American Public Health Association® (APHA). The oldest and largest organization of public health professionals in the world, APHA represents approximately 30 000 members from more than 50 occupations of public health.

Submissions: Visit www.editorialmanager.com/ajph or ajph.edmgr.com for online manuscript preparation and submission guidelines. Contributions of original unpublished research, social science analyses, scholarly essays, critical commentaries, departments, and letters to the editor are welcome. Questions? Write ajph.submissions@apha.org or call APHA at (202) 777-2469.

Print plus online subscriptions: Institutional price (print copy with online access for a single institution and all authorized users, regardless of geographic location) varies by size of organization and ranges from $993–$1445 for US organizations, and $1073–$1526 for international organizations (air delivery); multiple campuses not permitted without special arrangement. Details of the tiered pricing system at https://subscriptionoffice.com/pages/apha-landing-page. To order, write apha.subscriptions@apha.org.

Online-only subscriptions: Institutional price for one institution and its authorized users (regardless of geographic location) is $878–$1307. To order, write apha.subscriptions@apha.org. For academic consortia or multisite corporate subscriptions, contact apha.subscriptions@apha.org.

Print-only subscriptions: Institutional price is US $701, $782 international.

Back print issues: A limited number of print issues are for sale. Single copies are US $49, $55 international (air delivery). Shipping included; prepay only. To order, write apha.subscriptions@apha.org.

Reprints: For prices and ordering information on 50 or more reprints, check the Reprints section at www.ajph.org. To order smaller quantities of reprints (rush delivery), use the "Purchase Article" link on the article site itself.

Electronic access: Online articles more than 10 years old are available free for personal use at www.ajph.org. Recent articles are available through pay-per-view: single PDF article for $24, single issue access for 24 hours for $33, or entire site access for 24 hours for $38.

Postal information: Periodicals postage paid at Washington, DC, and additional mailing offices. Postmaster: Send address changes to American Journal of Public Health, 800 I St NW, Washington, DC 20001-3710.

Address changes: Send to AJPH, Membership Department (members) or AJPH Subscriptions (subscribers), APHA, 800 I St NW, Washington, DC 20001-3710. Or write to membership.mail@apha. org (members) or apha.subscriptions@apha.org (subscribers).

Indexes: Publications that index or abstract articles from AJPH include the following: Ageline, Asia (Applied Social Science Index and Abstracts), Biological Abstracts, Chemical Abstracts, CINAHL, Criminal Justice Abstracts, EMBASE, EMCare, Environmental Abstracts, e-psyche, ERIC, ETOH (Alcohol and Alcohol Problems Science Database), Excerpta Medica, Food Science and Technology, General Science Index, Grateful Med, Hospital Literature Index, Human Resources Abstracts, International Pharmaceutical Abstracts (IPA), Medline, Physical Education Index, Pollution Abstracts, Psychological Abstracts, PsychINFO, Safety Science Abstracts, Sage Family Studies Abstracts, Sage Human Resources Abstracts, Science Citation Index, SCOPUS, SIIC Data Bases, Social Work Research and Abstracts, and Statistical Reference Index (SRI)/LexisNexis.

AJPH

A PUBLICATION OF THE
AMERICAN PUBLIC HEALTH ASSOCIATION

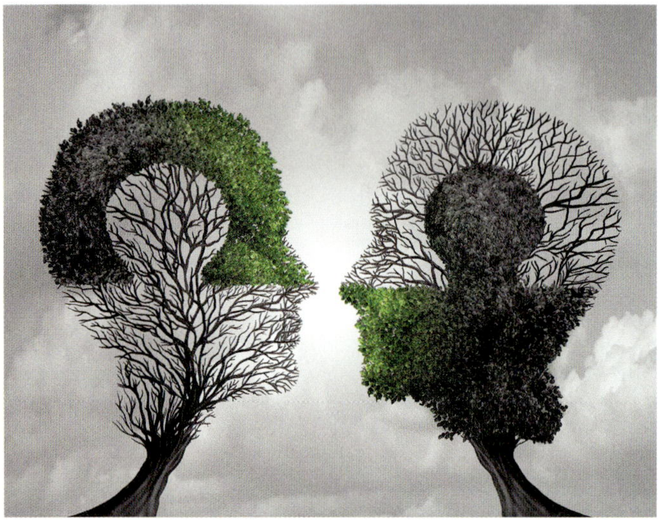

COVER: Teaming up for public health action among groups with differing viewpoints, values, ideologies, or perspectives has become more challenging – too many exist in bubbles. In this issue of *AJPH* we offer a new paradigm for expanding the notion of diversity to include diversity of thought and perspective from lived experiences.

Cover image and selection by Aleisha Kropf, Image Editor. Illustration by Lightspring/Shutterstock, printed with permission.

APHA
AMERICAN PUBLIC HEALTH ASSOCIATION
For science. For action. For health.

Promoting public health research, policy, practice, and education is the *AJPH* mission. As we widen our scope to embrace global issues, we also sharpen our focus to support the needs of public health practitioners. We invite contributions of original unpublished research, opinion and commentary, and letters to the editor.

The *Journal* is printed on acid-free recycled paper.

OPEN ACCESS | ONLINE ONLY | PODCAST | DATA SUPPLEMENT AVAILABLE

EDITOR'S CHOICE

1036 Public Health Common Ground: The Proof by COVID-19
A. Morabia

BOOKS & MEDIA

1037 US Supreme Court Doctrines in COVID-19 Cases Threaten Public Health
M. A. Rothstein

1040 Letting the Past Speak to the Present (and the Future)
K. Staub

OPINIONS, IDEAS, & PRACTICE

EDITORIALS

1043 Looking Back: Victimization of Transgender Persons and the Criminal Legal System
V. Baćak

1046 Policies Have Consequences: Measuring Excess Deaths During the COVID-19 Pandemic
S. H. Woolf

1050 Looking Back: Comment on "Economic Crisis, Restrictive Policies, and the Population's Health and Health Care: The Greek Case"
S. Galea

1053 Climate Justice and Health Equity: A Public Health of Consequence, October 2023
F. Kapadia

PERSPECTIVES

1055 Translational Bioethics and Public Health
M. A. Rothstein

1059 Indigenous Peoples and Cultural Safety in Public Health
M. Carlson and N. Redvers

1064 Teaching Systems Thinking as a Foundational Public Health Competency Can Be Improved
L. Paina and J. Glenn

1068 The Abortion Double Bind
D. Fox

1074 Unpacking Cochrane's Update on Masks and COVID-19
B. M. Gurbaxani, A. N. Hill, and P. Patel

1079 Power Up: A Call for Public Health to Recognize, Analyze, and Shift the Balance in Power Relations to Advance Health and Racial Equity
J. C. Heller, P. J. Fleming, R. J. Petteway, M. Givens, and K. M. Pollack Porter

1083 Time to End Racial Disparities in Buprenorphine Access
H. Rosen and C. O. Cunningham

NOTES FROM THE FIELD

1086 FORWARD: Building a Model to Hold Schools of Public Health Accountable for Antiracism Work
S. Garbers, M. A. Joseph, B. Jankunis, M. O'Brien, and L. P. Fried

1089 Integrated COVID-19 Interventions in a Native American Community: Arizona, December 25, 2021–January 31, 2022
E. A. Van Dyne, C. Jentoft, T. Boone, and R. M. Close

BUILDING COMMON GROUND

1093 On Building Common Ground: An *AJPH* Special Section
M. Fine, W. J. Kassler, and T. T. LeBlanc

1096 Quality and (Un)Certainty of Information: A Critical Concern for Building Common Ground
T. T. LeBlanc

1099 The Crosscurrents Dialogue Model: 2019–2023
R. H. Bernier

1102 Overcoming Public Health "Surveillance": When Words Matter
W. J. Kassler and C. L. Bowman

1106 I Hear You: Seeking Population Health Common Ground
S. Magnan and D. Kindig

1110 Building a "We" With Deliberative Dialogue in Pursuit of Health for All
E. Blacksher, Y. Asada, M. Danis, M. R. Gold, N. Kassebaum, and J. S. Onge

1114 Generation Z Challenges Partisan Divides for Health Equity
P. M. Alberti, K. Orgera, and C. S. Alvarado

RESEARCH & ANALYSIS

OPEN-THEMED RESEARCH

1116 Geographic and Socio-demographic Variations in Prevalence of Mental Health Symptoms Among US Youths, 2022
J. Liu, Z. Zhou, X. Cheng, and N. Vangeepuram

1120 Communities at Risk for Mpox and Stigmatizing Policies: A Randomized Survey, Republic of Korea, 2022
Y. Choi and A. M. Fox

BACKMATTER

ERRATA

1128 Erratum In: "Erratum In: 'Living Alone and Suicide Risk in the United States, 2008–2019'"

OTHER DEPARTMENTS

1136 Subscription Form

Public Health Common Ground: The Proof by COVID-19

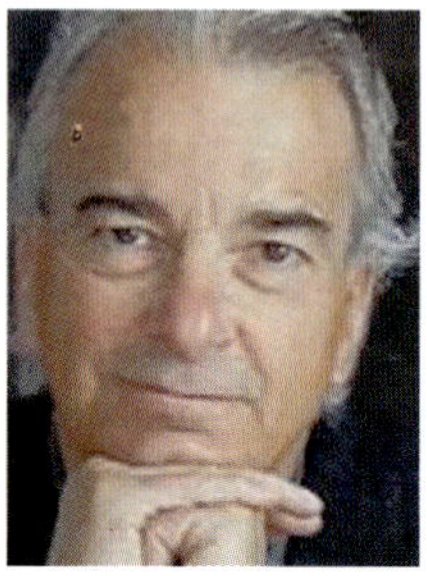

The theme of the *AJPH* special section "Building Common Ground," curated by associate editor Tanya Telfair LeBlanc and guest editors William Kassler and Michael Fine, is not novel for this journal. The idea is that people can team up and act together to improve public health even when different reasons motivate them.

In 2018, we began to promote the "public health dialogue" and invited points and counterpoints from experts with shared concerns but vastly different opinions about key issues, such as public health advocacy, the environment, health insurance, and structural racism (https://bit.ly/3Qf5CYa).

In 2020, pairs of public health professionals with different political leanings discussed issues such as vaccine hesitancy, the future of the Centers for Disease Control and Prevention (CDC), the 10 essential public health services, the future of state and local health departments, whether there is still a role for primary care, and the pathway to health care equity (https://bit.ly/3KfrQFu).

In 2021, the exchanges covered sensitive issues, such as racism and structural racism, gun violence prevention, single-payer health insurance, public health advocacy, the Environmental Protection Agency, and more (https://bit.ly/3OatBVx).

In 2023, we had different opinions expressed about what could be done to support pregnant persons following the 2022 decision of the US Supreme Court abrogating *Roe v Wade*: the federally protected right to abortion (https://bit.ly/3rLfMWa).

The public health response to COVID-19 has brought a new collection of evidence that, when the health of the public is at risk, public health personnel rally to act using the same strategies, such as mass vaccination in the case of COVID-19. It was quickly scientifically obvious that the vaccine saved lives and that older people were at greatest risk for morbidity and mortality from COVID-19. All US states rushed to vaccinate those aged 65 years and older. The national coverage was 97% (https://bit.ly/3Ki0FKe).

Even states that achieved the least coverage, Arkansas (83%) and Alabama (84%), made major efforts to protect their populations. The efforts were even greater than state averages suggest because these two states also have large fractions of their populations living in rural areas: Arkansas is 41% rural and Alabama is 44% rural (much more than California at 5%, Massachusetts at 8%, and New York at 12%; US Census, 2010). Consider urban areas where access to vaccination is easier: coverage in Little Rock (Pulaski County, AR) was 86% and in Birmingham (Jefferson County, AL) was 93%.

When it came to protecting older persons, there was no ideological polemic or political polarization. The job was just done. It could have been done better. It could have been done more equitably. But the numbers irrefutably show that the COVID-19 vaccination undertaking was a national effort that the public health leadership helped coordinate and achieve.

Also, public health progress cannot be assigned to a specific party: the Occupational Safety and Health Administration (Richard Nixon, R), the President's Emergency Plan for AIDS Relief (George W. Bush, R), the different parts of Medicare (Lyndon B. Johnson, D; George W. Bush, R), the Affordable Care Act (Barack Obama, D), the Environmental Protection Agency (Richard Nixon, R), and so on. Unfortunately, policymakers are sometimes united in degrading public health, as in the case of the weakening and marginalization of the CDC that has been evolving for decades across Republican and Democratic administrations.

Everyone contributing to *AJPH* agrees that disagreement should be overcome using current and historical evidence. Publishing such evidence is precisely the mission of *AJPH*. It is an attempt to link people of radically different political views who have in common a dedication to public health and an agreement that policy should be anchored as much as possible in objective bases. Dialoguing may sometimes be frustrating, but it enriches our understanding of how others live and think. It helps everyone to be more effective. AJPH

Alfredo Morabia, MD, PhD
Editor-in-Chief, AJPH
@AlfredoMorabia

DOI: https://doi.org/10.2105/AJPH.2023.307401

47 Years Ago

The Cigarette Smoking/Lung Cancer Hypothesis

The persistent controversy regarding the role of smoking in lung cancer cannot be resolved merely by escalating the force of arguments pro and con. . . . Study of the arguments from all sides reveals some common ground upon which we might proceed more dispassionately. While debating the relative *importance* of smoking, we, can, nevertheless, agree that cigarette smoking is at least *included* in the array of causal factors. A concern for appropriate public health policies and activities relevant to smoking and cancer follows from this agreement. Continued divisiveness around the precise contribution of smoking has potentially two tragic consequences for policy. On the one hand, to insist that smoking independently accounts for lung cancer is to construct an obstacle to future investigations and reappraisals of environmental carcinogens. On the other hand, there can be no question that widespread cessation of smoking would result in more good than harm. To dilute the importance of smoking is to foolishly divert us from an important goal.

From AJPH, *February 1976, pp. 132–133.*

53 Years Ago

Public Health and the Political Process—Lessons From the Passage of Medicaid

Though the APHA may differ with the other groups on certain matters, it is nonetheless urgent that specific effort be directed at building coalitions for specific public health measures wherever possible. To a much greater extent than in the past, public health must take the leadership to develop these alliances with diverse types of organizations, not only for research and training but also to develop health delivery programs. . . . Political strategy must be developed and potential allies sought. . . . It is interesting that in so many fields involving public-interest subjects, political strategy is left to the opposition. Does public health wish the AMA and its state and local counterparts, the chambers of commerce, or the commercial insurance industry, or even consumers to be the dominant voices on health and medical care? If not, what is public health doing to organize public health advocates?

From AJPH, *September 1970, p. 1697.*

US Supreme Court Doctrines in COVID-19 Cases Threaten Public Health

Mark A. Rothstein, JD

ABOUT THE AUTHOR

Mark A. Rothstein is with the Institute for Clinical and Translational Science, University of California, Irvine.

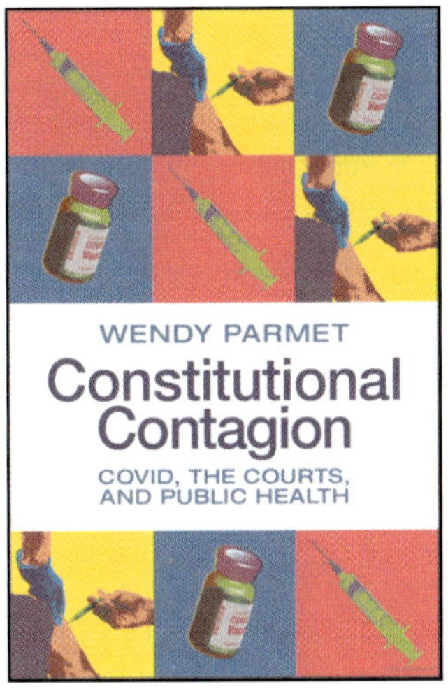

Constitutional Contagion: COVID, the Courts, and Public Health
By Wendy E. Parmet
Cambridge, UK: Cambridge University Press; 2023
248 pp; $24.99 (paperback), $75.00 (hardcover)
ISBN-10: 1009093835; ISBN-13: 978-1009093835

The mission of public health is to protect, preserve, and promote the health of the population. The challenge is to advance public health while also respecting such individual concerns as autonomy, privacy, and liberty in a diverse society. The conflict between population and individual interests also characterizes the inevitable legal disputes over public health policies, especially during public health emergencies. Historically, US courts have been highly deferential to reasonable and necessary public health measures to combat contagious diseases, even if they restrict individual liberties. That is no longer the case.

In her important and disquieting new book *Constitutional Contagion: COVID, the Courts, and Public Health*, Professor Wendy E. Parmet, JD, of Northeastern University reviews the history of constitutional law decisions on public health by the US Supreme Court and concludes that a series of COVID-19 era decisions markedly depart from longstanding and beneficial holdings, with dire consequences for public health.

The book's nine chapters include a discussion of *Roman Catholic Diocese of Brooklyn v Cuomo*,[1] the 2020 Supreme Court case in which the newly expanded conservative majority invalidated social distancing measures ordered by the State of New York (chapter 1); the principle of *salus populi suprema lex* ("the health of the people is the highest law"; chapter 2); the cases ending deferral to public health measures (chapter 3); the initial COVID-19 cases before the Supreme Court (chapter 4); the "negative liberty" rationale used in striking down mandatory masking and vaccination requirements (chapter 5); the lack of "positive liberty" public health protections (e.g., clean air and water; chapter 6); the unequal effects of the pandemic on minority and vulnerable groups (chapter 7); the deadly consequences of COVID-19 misinformation (chapter 8); and the politics of the pandemic (chapter 9). Each of these topics would justify a separate volume, but Parmet succeeds in weaving them together in a compelling, but depressing narrative.

To put the coverage of the book in context, in the US Constitution the previously independent colonies ceded certain limited powers to the new federal government, including foreign affairs and interstate commerce. All other powers not expressly given to the federal government remained with the states, including the "police power" to protect the health, safety, and morals of the people. That is why the states still have primary jurisdiction over public health.

The Bill of Rights granted individuals important liberties, including prohibiting the government from limiting freedom of speech, press, religion, and assembly and establishing the right to be free from unreasonable searches and seizures. These are considered negative rights because they restrict what the government may do. By contrast, the Constitution does not contain such positive rights as an individual right to education, health care, housing, or employment.

Parmet makes the tension between negative and positive rights and liberties a central focus of her book. I share my perspectives on some of the major themes explored in the book.

NEGATIVE LIBERTY

Constitutional contagion, the first part of the book's title, is described as "the prioritization of some conceptions of liberty over others in ways that endanger our health" (p. 221). The rationale for judicially favoring public health measures over individual liberties is eloquently captured by Justice John Marshall Harlan's famous 1905 opinion in *Jacobson v Massachusetts*, which upheld compulsory vaccination against smallpox: "There are manifold restraints to which every person is necessarily subject for the common good. On any other basis organized society could not exist with safety to its members."[2] Judicial deference to the exercise of police powers by the states, reluctance to second-guess public health experts, and recognition of the primacy of the common good characterized Supreme Court precedent for more than a century.

By late 2020, the newly dominant conservative bloc on the Supreme Court, including three new justices appointed by President Donald Trump, replaced common good with negative liberty as the driving force in deciding COVID-19 cases, primarily based on freedom of expression, religion, and bodily integrity. Although nonconformity and rugged individualism are cherished American values, prioritizing individual interests over the common good, especially during a pandemic, represents a grievous threat to public health.[3]

COVID-19 era judicial decisions have been especially deferential to claims of religious liberty in challenges to vaccination mandates, notwithstanding the fact that the leaders of virtually all major religions in the United States endorsed COVID-19 vaccination, including Catholics, Protestants, Mormons, Buddhists, Jews, and Muslims.[4] According to Pope Francis, being vaccinated was "the moral choice because it is about your life but also the lives of others."[5]

As a legal principle, religious liberty has never been absolute, and courts weigh it against other compelling interests, including public health. The duty to accommodate religion, based on First Amendment freedom of religion and statutory nondiscrimination provisions (e.g., Title VII of the 1964 Civil Rights Act, prohibiting employment discrimination), is not limited to established religions or dependent on specific religious doctrines. Although opposition to public health measures based on personal, political, or moral views is not in the ambit of religious liberty, many public officials and employers find it uncomfortable to interrogate individuals about the nature and sincerity of their beliefs and therefore grant religious exemptions from public health requirements.[6]

Irrespective of an individual's reason for opposing social distancing, masking, vaccination, and other measures necessary during a serious disease outbreak, public health experts have urged that the health of the population should take precedence over negative liberty claims.

MAJOR QUESTIONS

In the early part of the 20th century, the Supreme Court held that the authority of state and local governments to regulate public health was limited and did not extend to economic regulations, such as maximum work hours and child labor.[7] The Supreme Court abandoned this restrictive view of government power in a series of cases upholding congressional enactments during the New Deal. Courts consistently upheld federal and state laws regulating economic and public health issues if there was a constitutional basis for the enactment, such as the Commerce Clause, which gives the federal government the authority to regulate interstate commerce.

Furthermore, because of the increased complexity of regulatory matters, administrative agencies with technical expertise (e.g., US Food and Drug Administration, US Environmental Protection Agency) were authorized to clarify and implement statutory language, and courts upheld these regulations if they were reasonable and within the statutory delegation of authority. The Supreme Court stated that courts should defer to administrative agencies if the agency's interpretation of its enabling legislation was "not unreasonable."[8]

COVID-19 era Supreme Court decisions reversed course in striking down several public health regulations. In *Alabama Association of Realtors v Department of Health and Human Services*,[9] the Supreme Court invalidated a nationwide moratorium on evictions in counties with high levels of COVID-19 transmission in an effort to prevent further spread of the virus. Relying on the new "major questions doctrine," the majority opinion stated there was no evidence that Congress intended the Public Health Service Act to authorize the regulation of landlord–tenant relations. "We expect Congress to speak clearly when authorizing an agency to exercise powers of vast economic and political significance."[9]

Similarly, in *National Federation of Independent Business v Department of Labor*,[10] the Supreme Court struck down the Occupational Safety and Health Administration's emergency temporary standard for COVID-19, holding that the secretary of labor lacked the statutory authority to issue such a sweeping standard in the absence of an explicit congressional directive.[11] Thus, a statute specifically designed to protect occupational safety and health was deemed not to authorize regulating workplace exposures to a deadly virus that had already killed thousands of workers because transmission also occurred beyond the workplace.

The major questions doctrine, applied in these and other cases, represents extraordinary judicial activism that undermines the separation of powers and threatens to curtail an incomprehensibly broad range of government actions to protect public health.

IMPORTANCE OF PUBLIC HEALTH LAW

Alexis de Tocqueville's classic study, *Democracy in America*, was published in 1835. Among his keen observations about American life, he wrote, "There is almost no political question in the United States that is not resolved sooner or later into a judicial question."[12(p257)] Nearly two centuries later, this statement is even more apropos, especially as applied to public health. During the first 18 months of the COVID-19 pandemic, more than 1000 lawsuits were brought to challenge state and local public health actions.[13] There is little doubt that litigation will continue to play a pivotal role in nearly every public health issue for the foreseeable future, including abortion, contraception, childhood immunization, and responses to disease outbreaks.

For those immersed in public health law, Parmet's insightful scholarship provides an unparalleled history of doctrinal development, connecting the dots from the classic cases of the last century to the present. For nonlawyers, it may be a more challenging read, but it is worth the effort, and her analysis of the historical context and political implications of the cases rings true.

The book illustrates for all readers that public health measures are authorized by law, implemented pursuant to law, and constrained by law. For better or worse, the future of public health in the United States will depend not only on scientific advances and equitable access to essential public health measures but also on whether the courts rely on legal doctrines based on the common good or individual liberty. AJPH

CORRESPONDENCE

Correspondence should be sent to Mark A. Rothstein, 3787 Via Vuelta, Rancho Santa Fe, CA 92091 (e-mail: mark.rothstein@louisville.edu). Reprints can be ordered at https://ajph.org by clicking the "Reprints" link.

PUBLICATION INFORMATION

Full Citation: Rothstein MA. US Supreme Court doctrines in COVID-19 cases threaten public health. *Am J Public Health*. 2023;113(10): 1037–1039.

Acceptance Date: June 29, 2023.

DOI: https://doi.org/10.2105/AJPH.2023.307383

CONFLICTS OF INTEREST

The author has no conflicts of interest to declare.

REFERENCES

1. *Roman Catholic Diocese of Brooklyn v Cuomo*, 141 S. Ct. 63 (2020).
2. *Jacobson v Massachusetts*, 197 US 11, 26 (1905).
3. Rothstein MA. The coronavirus pandemic: public health and American values. *J Law Med Ethics.* 2020;48(2):354–359. https://doi.org/10.1177/1073110520935350
4. Rollins J. Where do major US religions stand on the COVID-19 vaccination? July 31, 2021. Available at: https://www.ksl.com/article/50211951/where-do-major-us-religions-stand-on-the-covid-19-vaccination. Accessed July 10, 2023.
5. McElwee JJ. Pope Francis suggests people have moral obligation to take coronavirus vaccine. National Catholic Reporter. January 11, 2021. Available at: https://www.ncronline.org/vatican/pope-francis-suggests-people-have-moral-obligation-take-coronavirus-vaccine. Accessed July 10, 2023.
6. Rothstein MA. COVID vaccine mandates and religious accommodation in employment. *Hastings Cent Rep.* 2021;52(1):8–9. https://doi.org/10.1002/hast.1294
7. *Lochner v New York*, 198 US 45 (1905).
8. *Chevron USA, Inc. v Natural Resources Defense Council*, 467 US 837 (1984).
9. *Alabama Association of Realtors v Department of Health and Human Services*, 141 S. Ct. 2485, 2489 (2021).
10. *National Federation of Independent Business v Occupational Safety and Health Administration*, 142 S. Ct. 661 (2022).
11. Rothstein MA. The OSHA COVID-19 case and the scope of the Occupational Safety and Health Act. *J Law Med Ethics.* 2022;50(2):368–374. https://doi.org/10.1017/jme.2022.64
12. Tocqueville A. *Democracy in America.* Mansfield HC, Winthrop D, trans. and eds. New York, NY: Harper Perennial Modern Classics; 2000.
13. Mellow MM, Parmet WE. Public health law after COVID-19. *N Engl J Med.* 2021;385(13):1153–1155. https://doi.org/10.1056/NEJMp2112193

Letting the Past Speak to the Present (and the Future)

Kaspar Staub, PhD

ABOUT THE AUTHOR

Kaspar Staub is with the Institute of Evolutionary Medicine, University of Zurich, Switzerland.

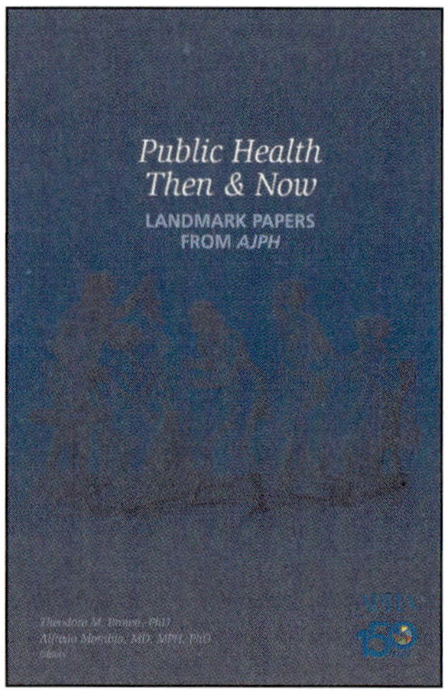

Public Health Then & Now: Landmark Papers From *AJPH*
By Theodore M. Brown and Alfredo Morabia
Washington, DC: American Public Health Association; 2022
600 pp.; nonmember price: $110.00, member price: $77.00
ISBN(s): 978-0875533261; 978-0875533278

The edited volume with its collection of articles reviewed here is a worthwhile reading journey through time and a multidimensional broadening of horizons. To commemorate the 150th anniversary of the American Public Health Association (APHA) in 2022, the association's official journal, *AJPH*, has published a special issue in the form of an edited book that presents 30 selected articles from *AJPH*'s "Public Health Then and Now" (PHTN) article category.

The beginnings of the PHTN section in *AJPH* date back to 1971, when George Rosen was editor-in-chief. Rosen emphasized the combination of historical and public health perspectives.[1] After Rosen's death in 1977, several generations of APHA leadership and the *AJPH* Editorial Board continued Rosen's mission.[2] Today, PHTN articles remain an essential feature of *AJPH*, contributing "fundamental perspectives on the past, present, and future of public health."[3(p2)] The primary motivation for the PHTN section is to provide a link between public health historians and practitioners and thus between "historical events and current public health realities."[3(p2)] PHTN articles are historical analyses of issues that have current relevance or can in some way be related to the present or the future.[2] Thus, PHTN articles are historical contextualizations of today's challenges, characteristics of past events, successes and failures, breaks and continuities, and similarities and differences between "then" and "now."

The book under review is edited by Theodore M. Brown and Alfredo Morabia (*AJPH*'s current editor-in-chief), who, as renowned experts in the history of public health and epidemiology, have decades of experience in these fields and thus embody the bridge between history and public health. From more than 350 PHTN articles published since the 1970s, the editors selected 30 landmark essays written by eminent experts in history, public health, or both. To make this selection, the editors each took the effort to reread all PHTN articles and then rate them according to their preferences. After reconciliation, they eliminated articles that covered similar topics. The articles finally selected are presented in order of their publication date. Although there is one article from the 1970s and two from the 1980s, most were published since the 1990s (up to and including 2019). The selected articles focus on the United States in the 20th century. The articles were only slightly modified and reprinted more or less in their original form.

A landmark, by definition, is an object that is easily seen from a distance and that allows someone to determine their location. Reading through the articles, it is immediately clear that, indeed, these landmark articles have been seen. If we take citations as a (limited) measure of visibility, the 30 selected articles bring together more than 3200 Google Scholar citations (as of June 2023). But visibility is of course much broader than citations, and impact is even harder to measure. I am convinced that these and many other PHTN articles have been read by thousands of public health scientists and practitioners or have been incorporated into teaching, thus influencing younger generations of public health professionals.

The selected articles are testimonies of their time—products of the period and the context in which they were written—not only in terms of the topics, concepts, and methods addressed but also in their argumentation and wording. In this sense, the articles themselves are quasihistorical sources. Each generation makes new historical assessments of the past. The timeless basis for this has been created in this impressive book by reproducing the articles in their original form. The past is left to speak for itself, and the interpretation is left to present and future readers, who will read these articles anew and differently as their distance from them increases.

In addition to the careful, diversified, and stimulating selection of articles, the main achievement of the two editors lies in their introduction, in which they map the 30 selected articles into major thematic areas and briefly summarize the main arguments of all the articles.[3] Because the editors' selections are one of the strengths of the book and should therefore be respected, this review will not highlight individual articles from the book in the sense of a further selection (all details can be found on the official Web site: https://ajph.aphapublications.org/doi/book/10.2105/9780875533278). Although the selected articles look back, the themes identified by the editors read like an agenda of contemporary major issues in public health:

- the relationship between public health and medicine (three articles),
- infectious diseases in a social context (e.g., tuberculosis, malaria, pandemics; six articles),
- chronic diseases (three articles),
- challenges to public health authority (four articles),
- addictions and harm reduction (three articles),
- occupational health (three articles),
- social labeling and racial and ethnic stigma (two articles),
- environmental challenges and opportunities (two articles),
- social movements and social critique (two articles), and
- data collection (two articles).

In the reviewer's opinion, this is a thematic panorama that does not leave many gaps with regard to the history of public health in the United States across the 20th century.

The selection of 30 articles is both the strength of the book and inevitably its only "limitation": the 30 selected articles represent only about 10% of all PHTN articles published to date. And the 90% of articles not in the book are no less worth reading. In addition, new PHTN articles are being published all the time. Interested readers will have to search for themselves to benefit from the full range of the PHTN treasury. Hopefully, as many public health professionals as possible will do so.

In public health, every new challenge is a mixture of what is already known and experienced, on the one hand, and what is new and surprising, on the other, in a context that may have changed. For the known part, it would be negligent not to draw on experience and experiential knowledge (that would be making the same mistakes over and over again). And also for the new and surprising part, it helps to have a toolbox of possible courses of action that can be adapted to the new context. The ability to draw on experience (both positive and negative) and thus on history (whether recent or distant) is, therefore, essential in the field of public health. And this experiential knowledge is acquired by professionals, institutions, and a field as a whole over decades of work and is passed on to subsequent generations.

But how does this knowledge transfer work in public health? Public health experts often report that there is a kind of trainee program in which experienced experts pass on their quasipersonalized experiential knowledge to younger colleagues. Then there is education and training, where it depends on how much importance teachers and curriculum developers attach to the inclusion of the historical perspective. On a more mediated and collective level, there are literature and data, which, thanks to the open access movement and increasing digitization, are becoming increasingly accessible, even retrospectively. Another possibility is public health journals that open the door to historical perspectives, for example with special sections. *AJPH*, with its PHTN section, has been a pioneer in this regard. And the book reviewed here is just another testimony to this vital commitment.

However, when it comes to bridging history and public health, too much still depends on interested individuals or editors. This connection should be more institutionalized, and more journals should follow *AJPH*'s lead to carry these bridges into the future. As history continues to be written, one can only hope that future editors of *AJPH* (and other journals) will keep the doors wide open to historical perspectives so that public health history continues to be heard and disseminated more often than just a little now and then. AJPH

CORRESPONDENCE

Correspondence should be sent to Kaspar Staub, Institute of Evolutionary Medicine, University of Zurich, Winterthurerstrasse 190, 8057 Zurich (e-mail: kaspar.staub@iem.uzh.ch). Reprints can be ordered at http://www.ajph.org by clicking the "Reprints" link.

PUBLICATION INFORMATION

Full Citation: Staub K. Letting the past speak to the present (and the future). *Am J Public Health.* 2023;113(10):1040–1042.

Acceptance Date: July 7, 2023.

DOI: https://doi.org/10.2105/AJPH.2023.307389

CONFLICTS OF INTEREST

The author has no conflicts of interest to disclose.

REFERENCES

1. Rosen G. The Committee of One Hundred on National Health and the campaign for a national health department, 1906–1912. *Am J Public Health.* 1972;62(2):261–263. https://doi.org/10.2105/AJPH.62.2.261
2. Yankauer A. An ongoing tradition. *Am J Public Health.* 1979;69(2):122. https://doi.org/10.2105/AJPH.69.2.122
3. Brown TM, Morabia A. Themes of public health history reflected in the *American Journal of Public Health*'s "Public Health Then and Now" essays. In: TM Brown, A Morabia, eds., *Public Health Then & Now: Landmark Papers From* AJPH. Washington, DC: American Public Health Association; 2022:1–20. https://doi.org/10.2105/9780875533278ch01

Looking Back: Victimization of Transgender Persons and the Criminal Legal System

Valerio Baćak, PhD

ABOUT THE AUTHOR

Valerio Baćak is with the School of Criminal Justice, Rutgers University-Newark, Newark, NJ.

Until 2016, the National Crime Victimization Survey (NCVS) lacked adequate data on gender identity, a prerequisite for measuring and understanding the victimization of transgender persons. The measure newly introduced in that year asked about sex assigned at birth and offered transgender as a response option to the question about gender identity. Although there continues to be no measure of nonbinary identity and transgender persons appear to be undercounted in the NCVS,[1] this is a major improvement. In their analysis, Flores et al.[2] were the first to leverage the newly available measure by pooling the 2017–2018 NCVS data, and they described rates of personal and household victimization of transgender persons nationally.

Given the quality and the weight of the NCVS in academic and policy conversations around crime and public safety, the study by Flores et al. was timely and valuable. They found that transgender persons reported personal victimization at a rate four times higher than cisgender individuals and twice the rate of household property victimization. Only about half of victimizations were reported to law enforcement. These findings will serve as a springboard as I highlight the endemic victimization of transgender persons in and by the criminal legal system ostensibly designed to provide them, like all citizens, with protection and safety.

According to national estimates from the 2011–2012 National Inmate Survey, the largest-ever survey of incarcerated individuals in the United States, 40% of transgender persons incarcerated in state and federal prisons have been sexually victimized over the past year (or since admission to the facility, if they were incarcerated for < 12 months) by another incarcerated person or facility staff member, as compared with 4% of their cisgender counterparts.[3] This disparity in the prevalence of victimization is many times higher than the disparity in the NCVS community-based sample reported by Flores et al.[2] In jails, sexual victimization of transgender persons was estimated at 27%, in comparison with slightly more than 3% among cisgender persons.

In community samples, rates of victimization are high but much lower than in jails and prisons. The largest and most reliable source of self-reported data on transgender persons in the community is the 2015 US Transgender Survey.[4] Among the survey participants who reported having been incarcerated in jail, prison, or juvenile detention in the year preceding the survey, 20% were sexually assaulted by facility staff or other incarcerated individuals, and 23% were assaulted physically. When asked about victimization in the community, 13% reported having been physically attacked in the past year, whereas 10% were assaulted sexually. Rates are consistently higher among transgender persons of color and those involved in the underground economy.

These figures unequivocally depict American jails and prisons as much more dangerous spaces than the community. Yet, institutions of the criminal legal system increase the risk of victimization in the community as well, as police and other law enforcement agencies engage in practices similar to those that take place inside jails and prisons.[5]

In the US Transgender Survey sample of 27 715 participants, 40% reported having interacted with police or other law enforcement officers in the past year.[4] Of these participants, 58% (who also reported that officers thought or knew they were transgender) reported mistreatment or harassment by police, ranging from misgendering to sexual assault. Furthermore, 57% of the participants reported that they were somewhat or very uncomfortable asking the police for help if they needed help. One third of Black transgender women who interacted with law enforcement officers who thought or knew they were transgender reported that officers assumed they were sex workers.

These findings are devastating for public health in general and transgender health specifically. Because of high rates of bias-motivated violence, discrimination, and barriers in accessing adequate health care, transgender persons are at an increased risk of poor mental health.[6] At the same time, incarcerated persons with psychiatric disorders are at higher risk of being victims of crime and suicide inside jails and prisons.[7] It is for these reasons that the transgender population depends perhaps more than any other population on protection and care while incarcerated, yet it appears to receive the least of both. Even though prisons are the only places with a legal mandate to provide health care, they are notorious for delivering substandard care, and this is especially the case for transgender persons, who rarely have access to gender-affirming treatments by adequately trained medical personnel.[8]

Victimization in jails and prisons also has consequences for recidivism by reducing the ability of formerly incarcerated individuals to successfully reintegrate into the community after serving time behind bars.[7] It entraps transgender persons in the revolving door of incarceration as they contend with the weight of trauma and associated psychological distress, often left untreated because of low rates of health care coverage[9] in comparison with cisgender individuals. Transgender persons may also avoid medical settings, where they are often exposed to prejudice, disrespectful behavior, and inadequately trained medical professionals, among other barriers.[6]

Moreover, victimization and neglect send a political message when violence is motivated by hate or bias and when it predominantly takes place in public institutions. The message loudly conveys that the lives of transgender persons and their status as citizens in a democratic society matter less. It should thus be no surprise that transgender victims avoid seeking help from public institutions essential to their well-being, whether law enforcement institutions or hospitals.[10]

In addition to the physical victimization examined by Flores et al., transgender persons are exposed to less obvious and insidious forms of institutional mistreatment that underlie individual acts of bias-motivated violence. The role of the criminal legal system must be considered more broadly within what sociologists have described as legal violence, "the normalized but cumulatively injurious effects of the law."[11(p1380)] In a similar vein, law professor Dean Spade used the term administrative violence to describe the harmful impact of "purportedly banal and innocuous daily administration of programs, policies, and institutions."[12(p73)] Although these forms of violence cannot be easily measured, their effects are wide-ranging and profound, and without them more obvious forms of physical and psychological violence would be much less likely. We must invest in research agendas that consider these institutional and individual forms of violence as connected and mutually dependent.

A consequential instance in which administrative violence meets physical force is at the point of gender classification in jails and prisons; this is where administrative violence sets the stage for other forms of violence.[12] Most jails and prisons assign incarcerated transgender persons according to sex assigned at birth.[13] This practice continues despite the 2003 Prison Rape Elimination Act guidelines, which stipulate that housing and programming decisions involving transgender and intersex persons cannot be based solely on genital status and that facility staff must give serious consideration to the individuals' views regarding their safety. Implementation of these guidelines is rare and falls far short of protecting incarcerated transgender persons. The continuing practice of assigning transgender persons to housing facilities on the basis of external genitalia or sex assigned at birth has horrific consequences.[14] A study in California showed that the prevalence of sexual assault among transgender women housed in a prison for men was 13 times greater than the rate among cisgender men.[15]

But even if gender classification and housing decisions in jails and prisons start to change, that can only be a relatively small step forward. These institutions will continue to be infused with harmful and consequential binary conceptions of gender and sexuality that devalue individuals who do not fit dominant norms around what it means to be a man or a woman. These practices are especially harmful to poor and Black transgender persons who have to contend with the intersecting disadvantage of transphobia and structural racism inherent to carceral institutions.[8]

This violence takes place in a country where the incarceration rate among transgender persons is at least twice the rate of incarceration in the general population and several times higher among poor and transgender persons of color.[4] With this context in mind and the staggering rates of violence that clearly show how jails and prisons make transgender persons even less safe than in the community, we must ask whether incarceration constitutes cruel and unusual punishment that violates their fundamental human rights. As there continues to be no structural change and little accountability for institutions that expose transgender lives to extreme rates of social suffering, is it reasonable to expect that the same system will create and enforce fair and effective solutions to the crisis of its own making? AJPH

CORRESPONDENCE

Correspondence should be sent to Valerio Baćak, PhD, Rutgers University-Newark, School of Criminal Justice, 123 Washington St, Newark, NJ 07102-3094 (e-mail: valerio.bacak@rutgers.edu). Reprints can be ordered at http://www.ajph.org by clicking the "Reprints" link.

PUBLICATION INFORMATION

Full Citation: Baćak V. Looking back: victimization of transgender persons and the criminal legal system. *Am J Public Health*. 2023;113(10): 1043–1045.

Acceptance Date: July 10, 2023.

DOI: https://doi.org/10.2105/AJPH.2023.307393

ACKNOWLEDGMENTS

I thank kristen kendrick, Jody Miller, Max Osborn, and Vanessa Panfil for valuable comments on the original version of the article and Katherine Bright and Lauren Wilson for research collaborations that helped shape the ideas presented here.

CONFLICTS OF INTEREST

The author declares no conflicts of interest.

REFERENCES

1. Brown A. About 5% of young adults in the US say their gender is different from their sex assigned at birth. Available at: https://www.pewresearch.org/short-reads/2022/06/07/about-5-of-young-adults-in-the-u-s-say-their-gender-is-different-from-their-sex-assigned-at-birth. Accessed June 13, 2023.
2. Flores AR, Meyer IH, Langton L, Herman JL. Gender identity disparities in criminal victimization: National Crime Victimization Survey, 2017–2018. *Am J Public Health*. 2021;111(4):726–729. https://doi.org/10.2105/AJPH.2020.306099
3. Beck AJ, Merzofsky M, Caspar R, Krebs C. *Sexual Victimization in Prisons and Jails Reported by Inmates, 2011–12*. Washington, DC: US Department of Justice; 2013.
4. James SE, Herman JL, Rankin S, Keisling M, Mottet L, Anafi M. *The Report of the 2015 US Transgender Survey*. Washington, DC: National Center for Transgender Equality; 2016.
5. Ritchie AJ. *Invisible No More: Police Violence against Black Women and Women of Color*. Boston, MA: Beacon Press; 2017.
6. Hsieh N, Shuster SM. Health and health care of sexual and gender minorities. *J Health Soc Behav*. 2021;62(3):318–333. https://doi.org/10.1177/00221465211016436
7. Schnittker J, Massoglia M, Uggen C. *Prisons and Health in the Age of Mass Incarceration*. New York, NY: Oxford University Press; 2022.
8. Baćak V, Thurman K, Eyer K, et al. Incarceration as a health determinant for sexual orientation and gender minority persons. *Am J Public Health*. 2018;108(8):994–999. https://doi.org/10.2105/AJPH.2018.304500
9. Bolibol A, Buchmueller TC, Lewis B, Miller S. Health insurance coverage and access to care among LGBT adults, 2013–19: study examines health insurance and access to care among LGBT adults. *Health Aff (Millwood)*. 2023; 42(6):858–865. https://doi.org/10.1377/hlthaff.2022.01493
10. Wirtz AL, Poteat TC, Malik M, Glass N. Gender-based violence against transgender people in the United States: a call for research and programming. *Trauma Violence Abuse*. 2020;21(2): 227–241. https://doi.org/10.1177/1524838018757749
11. Menjívar C, Abrego LJ. Legal violence: immigration law and the lives of Central American immigrants. *Am J Sociol*. 2012;117(5):1380–1421. https://doi.org/10.1086/663575
12. Spade D. *Normal Life: Administrative Violence, Critical Trans Politics, and the Limits of Law*. Durham, NC: Duke University Press; 2015.
13. Malkin ML, DeJong C. Protections for transgender inmates under PREA: a comparison of state correctional policies in the United States. *Sex Res Soc Policy*. 2019;16(4):393–407. https://doi.org/10.1007/s13178-018-0354-9
14. Ledesma E, Ford CL. Health implications of housing assignments for incarcerated transgender women. *Am J Public Health*. 2020;110(5):650–654. https://doi.org/10.2105/AJPH.2020.305565
15. Jenness V, Maxson CL, Matsuda KN, Sumner JM. *Violence in California Correctional Facilities: An Empirical Examination of Sexual Assault*. Irvine, CA: Center for Evidence-Based Corrections, University of California, Irvine; 2007.

Policies Have Consequences: Measuring Excess Deaths During the COVID-19 Pandemic

Steven H. Woolf, MD, MPH

ABOUT THE AUTHOR

Steven H. Woolf is with the Center on Society and Health and the Department of Family Medicine, Virginia Commonwealth University, Richmond.

AJPH October 2023, Vol 113, No. 10

On September 20, 2017, Hurricane Maria, a category 5 hurricane, swept through Puerto Rico. Official reports claimed that 67 people had died, but experts worried that the storm might have claimed far more lives. Researchers turned to an established epidemiologic tool, the measurement of excess deaths, to address these concerns. The term *excess deaths* refers to the difference between observed deaths from all causes and the number that would be expected under normal circumstances. In the case of Hurricane Maria, excess death calculations revealed that the storm had actually claimed more than 1200 lives.[1]

EXCESS DEATHS DURING THE COVID-19 PANDEMIC

The COVID-19 pandemic also raised fears of uncounted deaths, almost as soon as its virulence and lethality became apparent in spring 2020. The multisystem organ damage produced by the virus was not immediately clear to physicians, who first considered it a respiratory illness. Medical examiners used inconsistent methods to code causes of death. Concerns arose that some proportion of deaths attributed to other causes, such as heart disease or stroke, might have been miscoded COVID-19 deaths.

In addition to uncounted COVID-19 deaths, an increase in non–COVID-19 deaths was expected. Patients with life-threatening emergencies (e.g., unstable angina) were hesitant or unable to receive acute care, those with chronic illnesses often lacked access to providers or prescription medications, and acute psychological stresses induced by the pandemic, lockdowns, and socioeconomic upheaval precipitated fatal behavioral health crises (e.g., suicides, drug overdoses).

Excess death studies were launched around the world to quantify the number of uncounted deaths, and they immediately demonstrated that the pandemic was claiming more lives than news accounts suggested. In the United States, the Centers for Disease Control and Prevention (CDC) began reporting weekly death counts. The CDC also posted historical data on death counts for the same weeks in previous years, enabling researchers to model normal seasonal variation during prepandemic years and to use this benchmark of expected deaths to calculate excess deaths during the pandemic.[2–4]

The results were striking. For example, in an analysis published in this journal, Tatar et al.[5] estimated that total deaths in Florida during March to September 2020 were 15.5% higher than historical norms. Other studies reported that deaths were 20% to 40% higher than normal.[2–4] Explanations for the sizable gap included (1) uncounted or miscoded COVID-19 deaths in which the role of the virus was undocumented, or (2) deaths among people without COVID-19 who died from other causes because of complications induced by the pandemic, such as delayed access to care or emotional distress. (Conspiracy theorists—citing dubious evidence—claimed that the gap reflected deliberate underreporting of deaths to downplay COVID-19 or the alleged dangers of lockdowns, vaccines, or masks.)

LESSONS LEARNED

A strength of excess death calculations is their objectivity. Deaths are a hard metric; they transcend debates about how causes of death are coded. During the pandemic, researchers could estimate the number of excess deaths with confidence, even when the precise causes of these deaths had yet to be clarified. The same was true for studies of all-cause mortality or life expectancy, metrics that were also agnostic to cause-of-death attribution. During the COVID-19 pandemic, all these studies—those examining excess deaths, all-cause mortality, and life expectancy—sounded the same warning: the United States was experiencing a massive death toll that was larger than widely believed, highly racialized, and far greater than losses in other high-income countries.[6–8]

Sadly, racialized health outcomes are nothing new in the United States, but the inequities during the COVID-19 pandemic were particularly horrific. People of color were more likely to be frontline workers, live in low-income communities, and have limited access to care. They were more vulnerable to infection, complications, hospitalizations, and excess deaths and experienced enormous losses in life expectancy.[9] Decreases in life expectancy in 2020 were as high as 3.70 years and 3.22 years in Hispanic and non-Hispanic Black populations, respectively, compared with 1.38 years in the non-Hispanic White population.[6]

The heavy death toll among people of color drew public attention to long-standing racial/ethnic inequities and the legacy of systemic racism, and it came at an interesting time. The George Floyd murder occurred in May 2020, soon after the pandemic began, unleashing a summer of social unrest and public outcry for meaningful systemic change. The moment energized nationwide antiracism initiatives but also incited a backlash from an increasingly hostile White supremacy movement.

The pandemic also drew international attention to the poor performance of the United States, arguably the richest country in the world. This too was nothing new. For decades, the United States has had a "health disadvantage": Americans experience shorter lives and poorer health than people in other high-income nations, and the problem has worsened over time.[10] The disadvantage is not for lack of spending on health care, at which the United States excels, nor can it be blamed on singular causes such as obesity, opioids, or guns, as the evidence indicates something more systemic is to blame. Among the potential explanations are deficiencies in health care and public health services, a higher prevalence of unhealthy and risky behaviors, greater socioeconomic precarity, harmful physical and social environmental factors, and—at the macrostructural level—policies and social values that adversely affect downstream determinants of health.

HOW STATES CONTRIBUTED TO EXCESS DEATHS

It is worth remembering that US health statistics are the product of 50 states. The COVID-19 pandemic offered a vivid reminder of the strong influence of state policies on health outcomes. The Constitution vests public health authority with the states, which have always made decisions on matters affecting health. Examples range from tobacco taxes and Medicaid expansion to speed limits, firearm legislation, and policies affecting the social determinants of health (e.g., minimum wage, earned income tax credits). Over time, the influence of state policy on health has deepened and states have become more politically polarized, resulting in a widening divergence in state health trajectories.[11] For example, the range in life expectancy among the 50 states has widened since the 1990s, partly because of divergent policy choices. Montez et al. demonstrated that states that embraced more conservative policy orientations experienced larger losses in life expectancy than those with more progressive orientations.[11]

State influence on health policy was illustrated vividly during the COVID-19 pandemic, when response plans divided sharply along party lines. Whereas "blue" states often adopted more proactive policies to reduce viral transmission, "red" states often challenged public health guidance and scientific data and resisted pandemic control measures, such as masking and vaccination mandates. The partisan divide created a macabre natural experiment in which the effects of state policy on death rates could be measured in real time in two groups of comparison states. The "control group," states that weakly embraced or discouraged pandemic control measures, experienced longer surges in excess deaths during the initial outbreak in 2020.[4] They also experienced more excess deaths in 2021, when COVID-19 variants placed unvaccinated individuals at heightened risk. For example, during the Delta variant surge in fall 2021, Florida experienced more than triple the number of excess deaths as New York, even though the states had similar population counts.[12]

One mystery about 2021 is why the non-Hispanic White population—which should have been at lower medical risk (and was so in 2020)—experienced a larger decrease in life expectancy in 2021 (1.0 year) than the high-risk Hispanic and non-Hispanic Black populations (0.2 year and 0.7 year, respectively).[13] Although research is needed to fully explain why this occurred, one possibility is that those who rejected COVID-19 vaccinations and public health guidance were more likely to be White. Some conservative politicians and social media stoked an ideological fervor that demonized public health and may have hardened resistance among some White people, potentially costing lives. Studies show that death

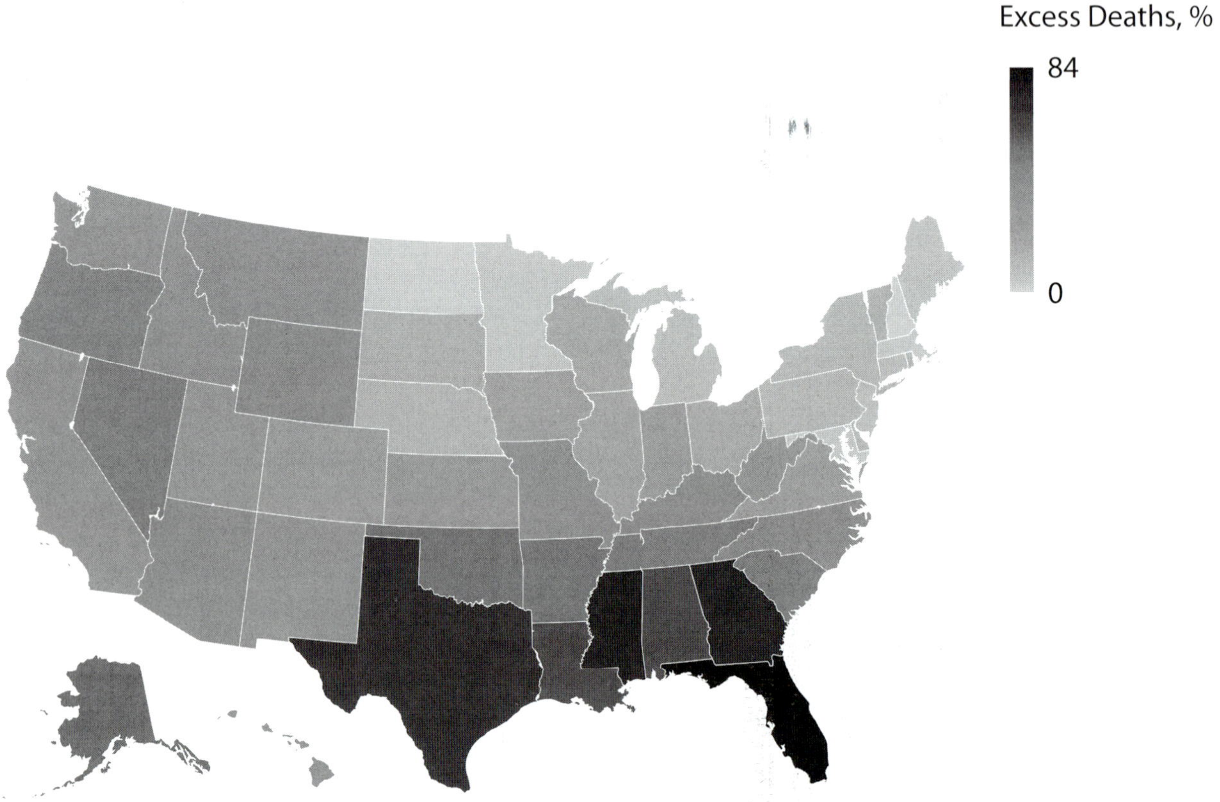

FIGURE 1— Percentage of Excess Deaths by State at Height of COVID-19 Delta Variant Surge: United States, Week Ending August 28, 2021

Source. Percentages calculated from excess death estimates from the Centers for Disease Control and Prevention, https://data.cdc.gov/NCHS/Excess-Deaths-Associated-with-COVID-19/xkkf-xrst, accessed July 4, 2023.

rates in 2021 were highest in states with Republican voting majorities and in rural counties, particularly in the South (Figure 1).[14,15]

The prospect of state policymakers putting lives at risk will not end with the COVID-19 pandemic. State legislation and court rulings that could adversely affect population health are sweeping the nation, notably those affecting women's reproductive health, LGBTQ (lesbian, gay, bisexual, transgender/-sexual, queer or questioning) rights, and transgender youths. These states are making it easier to own and carry firearms at a time when firearm-related deaths are increasing, easing regulations on industry and potentially reducing protections for workers and environmental health as the threat of climate change deepens, reducing the power of public health agencies, rolling back policies that promote the social determinants of health (e.g., social welfare programs), and resisting civil rights and antiracism reforms, if not challenging the very existence of racism.

While this is occurring, the US health disadvantage continues to worsen. As of 2021, more than 50 countries had achieved higher life expectancy than the United States—17 of them having done so for more than 50 years—demonstrating that it is possible for countries with far less wealth to protect the health of their populations.[10] What the United States lacks is not potential solutions but political will. Unless Americans get serious about protecting population health, studies of excess deaths will continue to deliver disappointing news. AJPH

CORRESPONDENCE

Correspondence should be sent to Steven H. Woolf, MD, MPH, Center on Society and Health, Virginia Commonwealth University School of Population Health, 830 East Main St., Suite 5035, Richmond, VA 23298-0212 (e-mail: steven.woolf@vcuhealth.org). Reprints can be ordered at http://www.ajph.org by clicking the "Reprints" link.

PUBLICATION INFORMATION

Full Citation: Woolf SH. Policies have consequences: measuring excess deaths during the COVID-19 pandemic. *Am J Public Health*. 2023;113(10):1046–1049.

Acceptance Date: July 7, 2023.

DOI: https://doi.org/10.2105/AJPH.2023.307390

CONFLICTS OF INTEREST

The author has no conflicts of interest to declare.

REFERENCES

1. Cruz-Cano R, Mead EL. Causes of excess deaths in Puerto Rico after Hurricane Maria: a time-series estimation. *Am J Public Health.* 2019;109(7):1050–1052. https://doi.org/10.2105/AJPH.2019.305015
2. Weinberger DM, Chen J, Cohen T, et al. Estimation of excess deaths associated with the COVID-19 pandemic in the United States, March to May 2020. *JAMA Intern Med.* 2020;180(10):1336–1344. https://doi.org/10.1001/jamainternmed.2020.3391
3. Centers for Disease Control and Prevention. Excess deaths associated with COVID-19, by age and race and ethnicity—United States, January 26–October 3, 2020. *MMWR Morb Mortal Wkly Rep.* 2020;69(42):1522–1527. https://doi.org/10.15585/mmwr.mm6942e2
4. Woolf SH, Chapman DA, Sabo RT, Zimmerman EB. Excess deaths from COVID-19 and other causes in the US, March 1, 2020, to January 2, 2021. *JAMA.* 2021;325(17):1786–1789. https://doi.org/10.1001/jama.2021.5199
5. Tatar M, Habibdoust A, Wilson FA. Analysis of excess deaths during the COVID-19 pandemic in the state of Florida. *Am J Public Health.* 2021;111(4):704–707. https://doi.org/10.2105/AJPH.2020.306130
6. Woolf SH, Masters RK, Aron LY. Changes in life expectancy between 2019 and 2020 in the US and 21 peer countries. *JAMA Netw Open.* 2022;5(4):e227067. https://doi.org/10.1001/jamanetworkopen.2022.7067
7. Islam N, Shkolnikov VM, Acosta RJ, et al. Excess deaths associated with COVID-19 pandemic in 2020: age and sex disaggregated time series analysis in 29 high income countries. *BMJ.* 2021;373(1137):n1137. https://doi.org/10.1136/bmj.n1137
8. Bilinski A, Thompson K, Emanuel E. COVID-19 and excess all-cause mortality in the US and 20 comparison countries, June 2021–March 2022. *JAMA.* 2023;329(1):92–94. https://doi.org/10.1001/jama.2022.21795
9. Shiels MS, Haque AT, Haozous EA, et al. Racial and ethnic disparities in excess deaths during the COVID-19 pandemic, March to December 2020. *Ann Intern Med.* 2021;174(12):1693–1699. https://doi.org/10.7326/M21-2134
10. Woolf SH. Falling behind: the growing gap in life expectancy between the United States and other countries, 1933–2021. *Am J Public Health.* 2023;113(9):970–980. https://doi.org/10.2105/AJPH.2023.307310
11. Montez JK, Beckfield J, Cooney JK, et al. US state policies, politics, and life expectancy. *Milbank Q.* 2020;98(3):668–699. https://doi.org/10.1111/1468-0009.12469
12. Woolf SH. The growing influence of state governments on population health in the United States. *JAMA.* 2022;327(14):1331–1332. https://doi.org/10.1001/jama.2022.3785
13. Arias E, Tejada-Vera B, Kochanek KD, Ahmad FB. Provisional life expectancy estimates for 2021. Vital Statistics Rapid Release. No 23. August 2022. Available at: https://www.cdc.gov/nchs/data/vsrr/vsrr023.pdf. Accessed August 3, 2023.
14. Bollyky TJ, Castro E, Aravkin AY, et al. Assessing COVID-19 pandemic policies and behaviours and their economic and educational trade-offs across US states from Jan 1, 2020, to July 31, 2022: an observational analysis. *Lancet.* 2023;401(10385):1341–1360. https://doi.org/10.1016/S0140-6736(23)00461-0
15. Paglino E, Lundberg DJ, Zhou Z, et al. Monthly excess mortality across counties in the United States during the COVID-19 pandemic, March 2020 to February 2022. *Sci Adv.* 2023;9(25):eadf9742. https://doi.org/10.1126/sciadv.adf9742

Looking Back: Comment on "Economic Crisis, Restrictive Policies, and the Population's Health and Health Care: The Greek Case"

Sandro Galea, MD, DrPH

ABOUT THE AUTHOR

Sandro Galea is with the School of Public Health, Boston University, Boston, MA.

AJPH October 2023, Vol 113, No. 10

How do we calculate, and place at the center of the public conversation, the return on investment of spending to protect human health? What is the role of nonhealth policymaking in preserving and elevating health? How do we avoid repeating cycles of health-adverse policymaking? The 2013 article by Kondilis et al., documenting the impact of the late-aughts economic crisis and attendant economic restructuring on population health in Greece, pushes us to consider the persistent and perhaps heightened importance of these questions, 10 years after the article was first published.

Kondilis et al. documented changes in health in Greece between 2007 and 2011.[1] The late-aughts global economic crisis severely affected the Greek economy, and Greece had to rely on loans from the International Monetary Fund (IMF) to finance the country's debt. The IMF loans came with conditions, including privatization of public enterprises and limits on public spending in sectors like health and education. Data by Kondilis et al. show how, coincident with these changes, a broad range of health indicators in Greece deteriorated. Suicide and homicide mortality, mental disorders, substance abuse, and infectious disease morbidity all worsened, and use of public inpatient and primary care services rose. A decade ago, this was a sentinel analysis showing the relationship between austerity economic policies and health.

The Greek data documented by Kondilis et al. are consistent with other data that illustrate how macro-level austerity economic policies are associated with poor health. Data from Russia, the Caribbean, and New York City show similar findings.[2–4] Conversely, data from countries in Latin America that went through economic crises without succumbing to austerity economic measures show that these countries did not have a commensurate downturn in health,[4,5] further suggesting a link between economic policies and health.

That macro-level economic policies affect the health of populations is not in any way surprising. Any number of conceptualizations of the role of social determinants of health consider upstream factors like economic and social policies as foundational to population health.[6,7] Canonical reasoning in the field, including the work of Geoffrey Rose, suggests that policies set the foundations for the production of health and can shift the distribution of health in populations.[8] Whereas investment in prohealth policies can result in improvements in health,[9] policies that limit social and economic achievement can harm health.[10] Revisiting this article by Kondilis et al. a decade after its writing is a reminder of the importance of documenting the consequences of economic changes on health, and of how little has changed in the past decade, despite knowing the impact of economic conditions on health. Their work highlights three important questions that may merit academic and public discussion, to the end of protecting human health from inevitable future economic crises.

SPENDING TO PROTECT HUMAN HEALTH

Our academic and public conversation about spending to protect human health is limited and halting, especially when we expand the scope to focus not only on the prevention or treatment of disease. Although we recognize that there is substantial spending on health and health care—including, for example, US annual health expenditures in excess of $4 trillion—we are much more constrained in thinking strategically about what we are willing to spend to preserve and protect health for longer-term consequences. The most recent example of this is the COVID-19 pandemic in the United States, which has cost the country an estimated $16 trillion, or roughly the annual GDP of China.[11] In no small part, the costs of COVID-19 reflect decades of underinvestment in public health and the resulting vulnerability to a previously unknown virus.[12] Similarly, austerity policies are driven in part by a perception that the cost of maintaining good health is too high, even though the cost of poor health is greater in the long term. A key challenge to our ability to countenance spending on health protection is that of time lags. Spending that is largely on medical care becomes "health" in the immediate present; we are spending on imaging machines that are used in the current year. Conversely, spending on public health, much as spending on social and economic infrastructure, can influence health many years down the road. This separates spending in the short term from the benefits that accrue in the long term. The time lag between spending and its consequences separates decision-makers, who have to make difficult decisions in the present, from the potential positive health benefits of their actions. Therefore, we remain limited in our critical thinking about return on investment from health spending, particularly when that return happens on a different time frame than our investment. This was the case during the Greek economic crisis and in the run-up to the COVID-19 pandemic, and it continues to be the case in the present postpandemic reality.

THE ROLE OF NONHEALTH POLICYMAKING IN PRESERVING HEALTH

The social, economic, and political determinants of the health agenda have become broadly established within public health thinking. It is now well understood that policies, urban environments, power, place, structural racism—all macro-level features of the world around us—influence the health of populations and, as such, should be part of the remit of anyone interested in population health and its application to the health of the public. A Health in All Policies approach is the operational manifestation of social determinants thinking, whereby we recognize that to promote health we need to think of and involve sectors—financial, housing, sanitation, law enforcement—that have not historically been seen as "health" sectors.[13] This recognition has implications both for those who are in the business of promoting health and for those who are in the nonhealth sectors. For the former, it means engaging with different sectors, including policymakers who are socialized to think rather differently, and encouraging them to see consequences of their actions through the lens of health. For the latter, it means making the effort to take on health as an outcome of interest in their deliberations. As the Greek economic crisis and similar case studies show, this is far easier said than done, particularly when coupled, as noted here, with time lags between actions of the nonhealth actors and results in health.[14] However, as this particular case shows, nonhealth sectors have an ineluctable role to play, and health cannot advance without their engagement. This puts the onus on health actors to engage counterparts in thinking about health, and to clarify, to nonhealth actors, the importance of having health as one of the key factors to be balanced in their thinking.

AVOIDING REPEATING CYCLES OF HEALTH-ADVERSE POLICYMAKING

This brings us to the third and perhaps most important implication of the Kondilis et al. analysis a decade later: how do we avoid future policymaking that puts health at risk? Recognizing both that protecting population health requires the engagement of nonhealth actors and that such engagement is difficult to do, particularly when the health benefits are temporally distant from the policy decisions, what are the levers that those in public health can use to mitigate the risk of repeated adverse-policy cycles?

Three thoughts might be helpful in this regard. First, greater and sharper clarity about the role of social and political factors in determining health is a helpful step toward diffusing these ideas. Not long ago, the notion that social factors mattered for health was relatively novel in medicine. That this is no longer the case is good, but it is also true that it has been widely accepted only in relatively recent years. The establishment of social determinants at the center of the health conversation is a necessary first step toward the broader communication of the role of such factors to nonhealth actors.

Second, those concerned with the health of populations need to become substantially better at telling the story of health. This story is still told principally through the lens of medicine, with narratives that center on individual clinicians healing individual, sick patients. Part of changing the public conversation will require better narratives about how investments in the prevention of disease and promotion of health and welfare are far preferable for societies, and well worth the cost.

Third, we need to highlight the moral and pragmatic need for nonhealth policies that advance health. This means empirical and expository scholarship that makes clear the essentialness of health as a human value, and the tremendous societal advantages of healthier populations. It will require this kind of scholarship to change the policy conversation, and to counter historical ideologies that have advanced austerity ideas without regard for their health consequences.

TEN YEARS AFTER THE ECONOMIC CRISIS

It is both sobering and motivating to revisit an analysis, 10 years later, that highlights the health consequences of economic crises, and to realize that such consequences would be the case today in another such crisis, much as we have seen after the recent pandemic. This should both sharpen our focus on investing in prohealth policies and energize the next generation of population health scholars to do the work that can shift the public conversation away from austerity economics once and for all. AJPH

CORRESPONDENCE

Correspondence should be sent to Sandro Galea, MD, DrPH, 715 Albany St, Boston, MA 02446 (e-mail: sgalea@bu.edu). Reprints can be ordered at http://www.ajph.org by clicking the "Reprints" link.

PUBLICATION INFORMATION

Full Citation: Galea S. Looking back: comment on "Economic Crisis, Restrictive Policies, and the Population's Health and Health Care: The Greek Case." *Am J Public Health*. 2023;113(10): 1050–1052.

Acceptance Date: July 18, 2023.

DOI: https://doi.org/10.2105/AJPH.2023.307394

ACKNOWLEDGMENTS

Thank you to Catalina Melendez Contreras for research assistance with this manuscript.

CONFLICTS OF INTEREST

The author has no conflicts of interest to disclose.

REFERENCES

1. Kondilis E, Giannakopoulos S, Gavana M, Ierodiakonou I, Waitzkin H, Benos A. Economic crisis, restrictive policies, and the population's health and health care: the Greek case. *Am J Public Health.* 2013;103(6):973–979. https://doi.org/10.2105/AJPH.2012.301126
2. Leyland AH. Alcohol, financial crisis and reform: learning from the Russian experience. *Eur J Public Health.* 2012;22(3):300. https://doi.org/10.1093/eurpub/cks051
3. Freudenberg N, Fahs M, Galea S, Greenberg A. The impact of New York City's 1975 fiscal crisis on the tuberculosis, HIV, and homicide syndemic. *Am J Public Health.* 2006;96(3):424–434. https://doi.org/10.2105/AJPH.2005.063511
4. Musgrove P. The economic crisis and its impact on health and health care in Latin America and the Caribbean. *Int J Health Serv.* 1987;17(3):411–441. https://doi.org/10.2190/7EC9-PM6N-6LLJ-X2PC
5. Waitzkin H. *Medicine and Public Health at the End of Empire.* New York, NY: Paradigm Publishers; 2011.
6. Wilkinson RG, Marmot MG. *Social Determinants of Health: The Solid Facts.* 2nd ed. World Health Organization, eds. Copenhagen, Denmark: WHO Regional Office for Europe; 2003.
7. US Dept of Health and Human Services, Office of Disease Prevention and Health Promotion. Social Determinants of Health. Healthy People 2030. Available at: https://health.gov/healthypeople/priority-areas/social-determinants-health. Accessed July 25, 2023.
8. Rose G, Khaw KT, Marmot M. *Rose's Strategy of Preventive Medicine: The Complete Original Text.* 2nd ed. Oxford, UK: Oxford University Press Inc; 2008. https://doi.org/10.1093/acprof:oso/9780192630971.001.0001
9. Langford R, Bonell CP, Jones HE, et al. The WHO Health Promoting School framework for improving the health and well-being of students and their academic achievement. *Cochrane Database Syst Rev.* 2014;(4):CD008958. https://doi.org/10.1002/14651858.CD008958.pub2
10. Meherali S, Punjani N, Louie-Poon S, et al. Mental health of children and adolescents amidst COVID-19 and past pandemics: a rapid systematic review. *Int J Environ Res Public Health.* 2021;18(7):3432. https://doi.org/10.3390/ijerph18073432
11. Cutler DM, Summers LH. The COVID-19 pandemic and the $16 trillion virus. *JAMA.* 2020;324(15):1495–1496. https://doi.org/10.1001/jama.2020.19759
12. Maani N, Galea S. COVID-19 and underinvestment in the public health infrastructure of the United States. *Milbank Q.* 2020;98(2):250–259. https://doi.org/10.1111/1468-0009.12463
13. Office of Policy, Performance, and Evaluation, Centers for Disease Control and Prevention. Health in All Policies. May 9, 2023. Available at: https://www.cdc.gov/policy/hiap/index.html. Accessed July 25, 2023.
14. Stuckler D, Basu S, Suhrcke M, Coutts A, McKee M. The public health effect of economic crises and alternative policy responses in Europe: an empirical analysis. *Lancet.* 2009;374(9686):315–323. https://doi.org/10.1016/S0140-6736(09)61124-7

Climate Justice and Health Equity: A Public Health of Consequence, October 2023

Farzana Kapadia, PhD, MPH

ABOUT THE AUTHOR

Farzana Kapadia is deputy editor of AJPH *and professor of epidemiology at the School of Global Public Health, New York University, New York, NY.*

The year 2023 may well be remembered for the multiple and intense climate crises that wreaked havoc across the world. From scorching heat domes that gripped the western and southern United States and major cities across the world to wildfires that burned large swaths of Canadian, European, and North American forests, these escalating climate crises are having devastating impacts on our environment and population. In this past year alone, the Northeast United States witnessed highly toxic air quality caused by forest fires in Canada, parts of Vermont experienced catastrophic flooding, and more tornadoes and hurricanes struck suburban and rural areas across the world. And as of this writing, the full extent of the devastation and loss of life from the wildfires that ravaged parts of Lahaina, Maui, an area that was formerly a wetland, is still being assessed. One common thread across these climate crises is that they will continue to bring more extreme weather and endanger our natural resources and physical spaces, in turn undermining any progress that has been made in reducing health inequities among vulnerable populations. Thus, among structurally marginalized people and communities—those who contribute the least to causing climate crises yet who are most often impacted first and worst—the need for actions that reduce the impact of climate crises is a matter not only of climate justice but also of reducing further health inequities.

In reviewing the evidence base in *AJPH* on the health impacts of climate crises, we see that they can be categorized into two collections. First is a collection on the numerous adverse health impacts resulting from climate crises. And a second collection includes a growing number of reports on action plans and behavioral modifications that can allow communities and individuals to adapt or prepare for climate crises.

HEALTH IMPACTS OF CLIMATE CRISES

In 2011, Knowlton et al. presented simulations of heat-related mortality in the Northeast. While their findings suggested that premature mortality among urban residents would increase with little attention to reducing the causes of climate change, they also predicted increases in premature mortality among suburban and rural areas.[1]

Fast-forward and simulations like that conducted by Knowlton et al. are no longer necessary. The immediate health impacts of climate crises are undeniable as a growing number of studies continue to document increased morbidity and mortality following catastrophic climate crises. Periods of excessive heat are linked to excess mortality among the elderly[2] as well as increased risk of infant mortality.[3] And this excess mortality, while initially thought to disproportionately affect persons residing in dense, urban areas,[4] also affects individuals in suburban and rural areas that lack infrastructure and resources to provide or support heat action plans (HAPs).[5]

The broader health-related impacts of excessive heat among vulnerable persons cannot be ignored. Excess temperatures are linked to increased hospitalizations among persons experiencing homelessness[6,7] as well as farmworkers,[8] both where they work and in the often-substandard housing they are made to reside in. In addition, a report examining poor air quality as a function of days of heavy wildfire smoke documented increased burden from wildfire smoke to have an impact on communities with a higher proportion of structurally marginalized and vulnerable people living in underresourced settings and at greater risk for respiratory and cardiac distress.[9] Climate crises intensify already existing health and social disparities in vulnerable communities, adding multiple and overlapping shocks—loss of housing and shelter as well as access to safe water and food—that further entrench people in poverty and widen health inequalities.

Finally, climate crises are associated with increases in unintentional and intentional injury-related deaths.[10] And in already vulnerable settings, where emergency services are already stretched thin, extreme heat events place an even greater burden on police, fire, and emergency services.[11]

ACTION PLANS FOR CLIMATE CRISES

In 2004, Bernard and McGeehin reported on their efforts to identify and review HAPs across major US cities; their

AJPH October 2023, Vol 113, No. 10

findings indicated either a lack of any planning or cursory plans to mitigate the health impacts of excessive heat.[12] Fast-forward to 2023, and Randazza et al. completed a review of HAPs representing 21 large cities and counties across the United States and representing seven of the 10 US Department of Health and Human Services administrative regions.[13] Their review suggests that HAPs can serve as templates for building strategies to facilitate cooperation across multiple agencies to mitigate the multilevel harms wrought by climate crises. However, their review also highlights key gaps that must be shored up to meet the needs of vulnerable groups that are often left behind but most often the hardest impacted by heat-related climate crises. Specifically, fostering greater outreach to and collaboration with community organizations serving vulnerable communities can build greater trust and understanding of how to manage during climate crises. In addition, providing information in multiple languages, as well as in multiple locations—in community-based organizations, places of worship, places of employment, etc.—can extend the reach as well as acceptability of information. Such efforts will yield greater impact in fostering resilience to climate crises in vulnerable populations and vulnerable settings.

CONCLUSION

Now is our time to fully and actively embrace a public health agenda that promotes comprehensive and equitable strategies to reduce the causes of climate crises and fight for environmental justice. These actions can no longer be sidelined if we seek to mitigate adverse health impacts and to slow the growing health inequities resulting from climate crises. While locally relevant and appropriate action plans will play a critical role in fostering greater resilience to climate threats, for the most vulnerable in our population, alone they are insufficient. Equally if not more necessary are the structural and societal changes that we clearly must make, and can no longer ignore, to prevent the continued rise of global temperatures. The United Nations Sustainable Development Goals (https://bit.ly/47pLHvJ) provide actions that we can take to reduce greenhouse gas emissions, prevent rising temperatures, and protect our air, water, and global home. And as evidenced by the August 2023 ruling in *Held v Montana* (https://bit.ly/3OM23WU), US courts are beginning to recognize the harmful impact of climate change on the constitutional right to "a clean and healthful environment." This legal challenge is one of many that tests US states' recognition of industry activities that continue to fuel climate crises as harmful to the health and well-being of its populations (https://bit.ly/3qSp7vd).

Living through the Anthropocene means that we are the first generation to bear witness to the devastation wrought by climate crises. It also means that we may be the last generation that has some hope for effecting the change we need. AJPH

CORRESPONDENCE

Correspondence should be sent to Farzana Kapadia, PhD, MPH, New York University, School of Global Public Health, 708 Broadway, Room 729, New York, NY 10003 (e-mail: farzana.kapadia@nyu.edu). Reprints can be ordered at https://ajph.org by clicking the "Reprints" link.

PUBLICATION INFORMATION

Full Citation: Kapadia F. Climate justice and health equity: a public health of consequence, October 2023. *Am J Public Health*. 2023;113(10):1053–1054.

Acceptance Date: July 24, 2023.

DOI: https://doi.org/10.2105/AJPH.2023.307404

CONFLICTS OF INTEREST

The author has no conflicts of interest to disclose.

REFERENCES

1. Knowlton K, Lynn B, Goldberg RA, et al. Projecting heat-related mortality impacts under a changing climate in the New York City region. *Am J Public Health*. 2007;97(11):2028–2034. https://doi.org/10.2105/AJPH.2006.102947
2. Kosatsky T, Henderson SB, Pollock SL. Shifts in mortality during a hot weather event in Vancouver, British Columbia: rapid assessment with case-only analysis. *Am J Public Health*. 2012;102(12):2367–2371. https://doi.org/10.2105/AJPH.2012.300670
3. Schinasi LH, Bloch JR, Melly S, Zhao Y, Moore K, De Roos AJ. High ambient temperature and infant mortality in Philadelphia, Pennsylvania: a case–crossover study. *Am J Public Health*. 2020;110(2):189–195. https://doi.org/10.2105/AJPH.2019.305442
4. Dang TN, Van DQ, Kusaka H, Seposo XT, Honda Y. Green space and deaths attributable to the urban heat island effect in Ho Chi Minh City. *Am J Public Health*. 2018;108(suppl 2):S137–S143. https://doi.org/10.2105/AJPH.2017.304123
5. O'Brien DT, Gridley B, Trlica A, Wang JA, Shrivastava A. Urban heat islets: street segments, land surface temperatures, and medical emergencies during heat advisories. *Am J Public Health*. 2020;110(7):e1–e8. https://doi.org/10.2105/AJPH.2020.305636
6. Schwarz L, Castillo EM, Chan TC, et al. Heat waves and emergency department visits among the homeless, San Diego, 2012–2019. *Am J Public Health*. 2022;112(1):98–106. https://doi.org/10.2105/AJPH.2021.306557
7. Hajat S, Sarran CE, Bezgrebelna M, Kidd SA. Ambient temperature and emergency hospital admissions in people experiencing homelessness: London, United Kingdom, 2011–2019. *Am J Public Health*. 2023;113(9):981–984. https://doi.org/10.2105/AJPH.2023.307351
8. Quandt SA, Wiggins MF, Chen H, Bischoff WE, Arcury TA. Heat index in migrant farmworker housing: implications for rest and recovery from work-related heat stress. *Am J Public Health*. 2013;103(8):e24–e26. https://doi.org/10.2105/AJPH.2012.301135
9. Vargo J, Lappe B, Mirabelli MC, Conlon KC. Social vulnerability in US communities affected by wildfire smoke, 2011 to 2021. *Am J Public Health*. 2023;113(7):759–767. https://doi.org/10.2105/AJPH.2023.307286
10. Casey JA, Parks RM, Bruckner TA, Gemmill A, Catalano R. Excess injury mortality in Washington State during the 2021 heat wave. *Am J Public Health*. 2023;113(6):657–660. https://doi.org/10.2105/AJPH.2023.307269
11. Williams AA, Allen JG, Catalano PJ, Buonocore JJ, Spengler JD. The influence of heat on daily police, medical, and fire dispatches in Boston, Massachusetts: relative risk and time-series analyses. *Am J Public Health*. 2020;110(5):662–668. https://doi.org/10.2105/AJPH.2019.305563
12. Bernard SM, McGeehin MA. Municipal heat wave response plans. *Am J Public Health*. 2004;94(9):1520–1522. https://doi.org/10.2105/AJPH.94.9.1520
13. Randazza JM, Hess JJ, Bostrom A, et al. Planning to reduce the health impacts of extreme heat: a content analysis of heat action plans in local United States jurisdictions. *Am J Public Health*. 2023;113(5):559–567. https://doi.org/10.2105/AJPH.2022.307217

Translational Bioethics and Public Health

Mark A. Rothstein, JD

ABOUT THE AUTHOR

Mark A. Rothstein is with the Institute for Clinical and Translational Science, University of California, Irvine.

Modern public health science and practice are characterized by innovation in such areas as prevention, surveillance, data analysis, policy development, and delivery of health services on a population level. Public health officials also need to respond to new scientific developments amid a crisis, as exemplified during the COVID-19 pandemic by efforts to vaccinate much of the population using novel mRNA-based vaccines. Translational bioethics, a type of research ethics, analyzes the societal implications of innovative scientific methods and discoveries with the goal of improving individual and public health. Although translational bioethics is designed to augment the ethics programs of National Institutes of Health (NIH)–funded translational science awardees, its emphasis on the societal implications of transformative research may be applied more broadly.

This article deals with three related concepts: translational research, translational science, and translational bioethics. Translational research involves scientific exploration using innovative techniques and technologies to expedite and enhance the development, testing, and implementation of diagnostics and therapeutics across human diseases and conditions.[1] Translational science is the systematic study of translational processes used to accelerate and increase the significance of research progressing from the bench to the bedside.[2] Translational bioethics, the focus of this article, analyzes the societal implications of novel scientific methods and discoveries. With the aims of translational research extending to adoption of innovative discoveries, it is appropriate for translational bioethics to consider the broader implications of the research, including policy analysis and development.

TRANSLATIONAL BIOETHICS

Since 2012, the National Center for Advancing Translational Sciences (NCATS) at the NIH has coordinated the translational science activities conducted or funded by the NIH.[3] NCATS also coordinates the efforts of 60 leading medical institutions funded to conduct research using translational science principles.

Research ethics is a required component of federally funded translational science grants, but, at present, this usually involves such traditional elements as the selection and recruitment of participants, balancing of risks and benefits, informed consent, and other criteria for institutional review board (IRB) approval. Although these issues are important, a narrow view of research ethics represents a missed opportunity. To parallel the ambitious, disruptive goals of translational science,[4] translational bioethics also should "address fundamental societal issues, including the effects of translational science on public health, health equity, and human flourishing."[5(p603)]

The customarily limited focus of research ethics is related to the regulatory process. The research regulations of the US Department of Health and Human Services ("Common Rule") explicitly prohibit IRBs from considering societal risks and implications of proposed research: "The IRB should not consider possible long-range effects of applying knowledge gained in the research (e.g., the possible effects of the research on public policy) as among those research risks that fall within the purview of its responsibility."[6] It would be necessary to revise the Common Rule to require IRB consideration of societal risks and benefits of proposed research.

Regardless of the federal regulations, IRBs are not well structured to consider broader societal issues because they often lack broad multidisciplinary perspectives and seek to produce reviews in a relatively short timeframe.[7] Presidential bioethics commissions, government entities such as the Office of Science and Technology Policy, and independent research organizations such as the National Academies of Science, Engineering, and Medicine could assess societal implications of innovative biomedical research. Nevertheless, there is merit in establishing wide-ranging bioethics assessments as part of the translational science process to take advantage of embedded, interdisciplinary collaboration and expertise. Importantly, the study of societal issues by institutions undertaking translational research should not be seen as preempting consideration of these often-complex issues by other entities and individuals. An unresolved issue is

AJPH October 2023, Vol 113, No. 10

whether translational bioethics programs should be funded by the NIH, individual research institutions, or some other source.

In briefly describing the substance of translational bioethics, a logical starting point would be the three common morality principles contained in the Belmont Report[8]—respect for persons (autonomy), beneficence, and justice—and their application to societal implications of innovative research.[9] As for autonomy, the balancing of individual and population interests is a foundational concern of public health ethics. Beneficence would assess the costs and benefits of innovative research on a societal level. Justice serves as the moral grounding for health equity, an essential principle in ethical implementation of health research.

The risks, benefits, and consequences of research on public health have been explored in other contexts by academics, practitioners, and public health officials with diverse professional backgrounds and perspectives. Translational bioethics, with its focus on the societal implications of translational research, is congruent with traditional public health ethics scholarship and policy development.

RESEARCH FUNDED BY THE NATIONAL INSTITUTES OF HEALTH

Translational bioethics, at least as envisioned as a part of the 60 academic medical institutions funded by NCATS at the NIH to conduct translational research, has four distinctive characteristics:

1. Integrated: Where appropriate, translational bioethics faculty and affiliated researchers (e.g., from social sciences and humanities) should work with translational scientists from the outset of new research undertakings. In collaboration with researchers, bioethics personnel should learn the goals, methods, and intended applications of the research; review the technical obstacles; ponder the societal risks, benefits, and challenges; and explore possible unintended consequences and long-term implications of the research.
2. Timely: By working with translational scientists, bioethics faculty and affiliated researchers are well situated to generate analyses of ongoing research activities, explore the societal challenges they present, and develop relevant policy options for clinical integration and public health. In many instances, the evaluation can take place much sooner than typical scholarly assessments of novel research, which often occur after a scientific publication or public disclosure of research findings.
3. Interdisciplinary and collaborative: Translational bioethics should be broadly interdisciplinary and, depending on the nature of the scientific research, could include the collaboration of experts with backgrounds in public health, humanities, social sciences, law, theology, and other disciplines. Individual bioethics scholars do not have expertise in all these areas, and, consequently, directors of translational bioethics programs should coordinate the efforts of a multidisciplinary team of investigators, as needed. For example, surveys, interviews, focus groups, and other methods can be used to explore public attitudes about ongoing research, including the views and concerns of diverse racial, ethnic, religious, and other groups. Because a single medical institution may not have all the necessary expertise, and because some issues are likely to arise in multiple research projects, collaborations among the NIH-funded clinical and translational science awardees should be developed.
4. Internally and externally oriented: In reviewing early-stage research design and implementation, bioethics personnel might identify concerns, such as privacy, economic consequences, or health equity, at a time when the research methodology can be modified more easily than would be possible at a later stage. Thus, the research itself might be improved by internal bioethics review. At the conclusion of the research, translational bioethics collaboration also could help identify the need for regulatory action, health education, health communication, or other externally directed strategies to inform policy development.

Translational bioethics should be constructive, collegial, and complementary. Its ultimate purpose should not be to discourage, delay, or defund research, but to advance the traditional research ethics principle of beneficence by minimizing risks and maximizing benefits, with an emphasis on societal issues. Nevertheless, translational bioethics scholars must be vigilant in maintaining their objectivity and independence from translational scientists. The credibility of any bioethical and policy perspectives developed would be seriously jeopardized by the perception or reality that bioethics faculty and affiliated researchers are subordinate to translational scientists or serve only to legitimize their research.[10] At the same time, embedded bioethics personnel must develop and maintain collegial relationships with translational researchers.

TRANSLATIONAL BIOETHICS IN PRACTICE

Conceptually, translational bioethics is extremely broad, and, therefore, assessments should be tailored to specific research. Some criteria for assessing translational research protocols and practices are the likelihood of success and significance of the research in advancing public health, the degree to which the research is likely to promote health equity, the projected economic and opportunity costs in implementing the research, the ease of integration of discoveries into the health care system, the public acceptability of the research, and the possibility of unintended consequences.

Translational bioethics programs linked to institutions funded to conduct translational science are similar in some respects to the Ethical, Legal, and Social Implications (ELSI) Research Program of the NIH.[11] Since the launch of the Human Genome Project in 1990, the ELSI program has funded numerous grants addressing the societal implications of genomic research, clinical genetics, and nonmedical applications of new technologies, such as DNA forensics. ELSI researchers are primarily funded by individual grants awarded and administered by the National Human Genome Research Institute.

Although the ELSI program is one model,[12] it has some drawbacks in the context of translational science. For example, separate research grants would lack continuity and integration with NCATS-funded research, and the process of obtaining grant funding likely would make the research process much longer than research conducted by embedded personnel. Other models also could be considered, including Belmont Report–type panels on various issues such as gene therapy and neural implants, and incorporating substantial public input.[13]

To be successful, translational bioethics programs need to be endorsed and supported by the NIH, institutional research administrators, and translational research investigators. Translational bioethics program leaders should approach their roles with humility and understand that multidisciplinary collaboration among and aside from NCATS-funded institutions is essential.

CASE STUDY: COVID-19

The recent experience with vaccines for COVID-19 illustrates how social and political factors can affect the uptake of novel public health interventions developed by Clinical and Translational Science Awards (CTSA)-supported or other researchers. At the height of the COVID-19 pandemic, when the first two mRNA vaccines received emergency use authorization from the Food and Drug Administration,[14] the public response varied widely. The hope and relief of public health officials and most of the public were met with ambivalence or outright hostility by a significant and vocal minority of the population.[15] The resulting, suboptimal vaccination rate led to an estimated 234 000 unnecessary deaths in the United States[16] and presented stark lessons to learn.[17]

Widespread vaccine hesitancy and refusal, however, should not have been a surprise. The United States has a long history of political divisions regarding public health interventions, including vaccination. For example, during the H1N1 influenza outbreak in 2009, millions of people refused vaccination, and millions of doses of vaccine had to be destroyed, with political party affiliation highly correlated with the likelihood of vaccination.[18]

Opponents of COVID-19 vaccination asserted libertarian arguments against coercive vaccine mandates, claims that the emergency use authorization was rushed, and even claims that the mRNA platform was genotoxic.[19] The technology used in the mRNA vaccines was developed over decades, and the COVID-19 vaccine was formulated and tested for the better part of a year.[20] This time period provided an opportunity for multidisciplinary research in psychology, sociology, political science, and other fields to consider possible personal, religious, and political objections.

It is debatable whether embedded bioethics analyses concurrent with vaccine development would have increased the uptake of the vaccine in the United States, but such an analysis and possible policy recommendations would have been justified by the gravity of the situation. With mRNA cancer vaccines and similar technologies on the horizon,[21] comparable issues undoubtedly will arise again.

The pandemic also presented numerous other important issues for translational bioethics assessments, including international cooperation in research to develop emergency preparedness strategies, open access to essential data such as genome sequences of emerging pathogens and epidemiological data, new surveillance measures such as wastewater studies, digital passports and other measures to monitor individual disease status, intellectual property laws and reimbursement policies on access to therapeutics, and a range of health equity issues—both domestically and globally. Although these vital issues have been and continue to be the subjects of ethical and policy analysis, integrating social sciences, humanities, bioethics, and public health policy with innovative translational science research is a strategy worth pursuing.

CONCLUSION

A major rationale for translational bioethics is recognition that scientific advances are not discovered, produced, and adopted in a vacuum. The value of even spectacular scientific discoveries is not self-evident to many nonscientists, and unintended negative social and economic consequences of innovative research are always possible. Individuals and institutions undertaking groundbreaking translational research have a moral obligation to support academically rigorous consideration of the societal implications of their research.

Translational bioethics aligns well with the traditional goals of public health ethics.[22] Although many questions remain about the funding, structure, and scope of translational bioethics, it has the potential to provide valuable, timely, multidisciplinary perspectives on significant societal issues. A highly beneficial outcome of translational bioethics programs would be aiding the seamless adoption and integration of impactful translational research that improves public health. AJPH

CORRESPONDENCE

Correspondence should be sent to Mark A. Rothstein, JD, 3787 Via Vuelta, Rancho Santa Fe, CA 92091 (e-mail: mark.rothstein@louisville.edu). Reprints can be ordered at https://ajph.org by clicking the “Reprints” link.

PUBLICATION INFORMATION

Full Citation: Rothstein MA. Translational bioethics and public health. *Am J Public Health*. 2023; 113(10):1055–1058.

Acceptance Date: June 3, 2023.

DOI: https://doi.org/10.2105/AJPH.2023.307362

ACKNOWLEDGMENTS

Kelly Carty Zimmerer provided excellent research assistance.

CONFLICTS OF INTEREST

The author has no conflicts of interest to declare.

REFERENCES

1. Austin CP. Opportunities and challenges in translational science. *Clin Transl Sci.* 2021;14(5):1629–1647. https://doi.org/10.1111/cts.13055
2. National Center for Advancing Translational Sciences. Translational science principles. Available at: https://ncats.nih.gov/training-education/translational-science-principles. Accessed April 18, 2023.
3. National Center for Advancing Translational Sciences. About the CTSA Program. Available at: https://ncats.nih.gov/ctsa/about. Accessed July 14, 2023.
4. Collins FS. Reengineering translational science: the time is right. *Sci Transl Med.* 2011;3(90): 90cm17. https://doi.org/10.1126/scitranslmed.3002747
5. Rothstein MA. Expanding the role of bioethics in translational science. *J Law Med Ethics.* 2022;50(3): 603–607. https://doi.org/10.1017/jme.2022.99
6. Department of Health and Human Services. Protection of Human Subjects. 45 CFR 46.111(a)(2) (2018).
7. Doerr M, Meeder S. Big data health research and group harms: the scope of IRB review. *Ethics Hum Res.* 2022;44(4):34–38. https://doi.org/10.1002/eahr.500130
8. National Commission for the Protection of Human Subjects of Biomedical and Behavioral Research. The Belmont Report. 1979. Available at: https://www.hhs.gov/ohrp/regulations-and-policy/belmont-report/read-the-belmont-report/index.html. Accessed April 23, 2023.
9. Beauchamp TL, Childress JF. *Principles of Biomedical Ethics.* 8th ed. New York, NY: Oxford University Press; 2019.
10. Rothstein MA. Translational bioethics and health privacy. *Ethics Hum Res.* 2023;45(3):40–44. https://doi.org/10.1002/eahr.500167
11. Meslin EM, Thomson EJ, Boyer JT. The ethical, legal, and social implications research program at the National Human Genome Research Institute. *Kennedy Inst Ethics J.* 1997;7(3):291–298. https://doi.org/10.1353/ken.1997.0025
12. Burke W, Appelbaum P, Dame L, et al. The translational potential of research on the ethical, legal and social implications of genomics. *Genet Med.* 2015;17(1):12–20. https://doi.org/10.1038/gim.2014.74
13. Evans JH. Translational bioethics and public input. *Ethics Hum Res.* 2023;45(4):35–39. https://doi.org/10.1002/eahr.500175.
14. Allen JD, Feng W, Corlin L, et al. Why are some people reluctant to be vaccinated for COVID-19? A cross-sectional study among US adults in May–June 2020. *Prev Med Rep.* 2021;24:101494. https://doi.org/10.1016/j.pmedr.2021.101494
15. Emery N, Dugerdil A, Flahault A. Vaccine hesitancies across the world in the era of COVID-19. *Am J Public Health.* 2022;112(11):1579–1581. https://doi.org/10.2105/AJPH.2022.307087
16. Amin K, Ortaliza J, Cox C, Michaud J, and Kates J. COVID-19 mortality preventable by vaccines. Peterson-KFF Health Systems Tracker. April 21, 2022. Available at: https://www.kff.org/coronavirus-covid-19/issue-brief/covid-19-continues-to-be-a-leading-cause-of-death-in-the-u-s. Accessed June 14, 2023.
17. Collins F, Adam S, Colvis C, et al. The NIH-led research response to COVID-19. *Science.* 2023; 379(6631):441–444. https://doi.org/10.1126/science.adf5167
18. Mesch GS, Schwirian KP. Confidence in government and vaccination willingness in the USA. *Health Promot Int.* 2015;30(2):213–221. https://doi.org/10.1093/heapro/dau094
19. ABC Fact Check. Anti-vaxxers say a new study claims mRNA vaccines can alter your DNA. Here's why that's bunkum. March 3, 2022. Available at: https://www.abc.net.au/news/2022-03-04/coronacheck-mrna-vaccines-not-genotoxic-pete-evans/100879220. Accessed April 18, 2023.
20. Dolgin E. The tangled history of mRNA vaccines. *Nature.* 2021;597(7876):318–324. https://doi.org/10.1038/d41586-021-02483-w
21. Fiedler K, Lazzaro S, Lutz J, Rauch S, Heidenreich R. mRNA cancer vaccines. *Recent Results Cancer Res.* 2016;209:61–85. https://doi.org/10.1007/978-3-319-42934-2_5
22. Bayer R, Fairchild AL. The genesis of public health ethics. *Bioethics.* 2004;18(6):473–492. https://doi.org/10.1111/j.1467-8519.2004.00412.x

Indigenous Peoples and Cultural Safety in Public Health

Megan Carlson, MPH, and Nicole Redvers, ND, MPH

ABOUT THE AUTHORS

Megan Carlson is with the Department of Population Health, School of Medicine and Health Sciences, University of North Dakota, Grand Forks. Nicole Redvers is with the Schulich School of Medicine and Dentistry, University of Western Ontario, London, ON, Canada.

There is a growing consciousness in the United States regarding the need to address structural root causes of health inequities for marginalized populations.[1] Addressing structural root causes are particularly imperative for Indigenous Peoples in the United States, who experience some of the highest rates of health inequities of any ethnic or racial group.[2] Public health (PH) literature has echoed the need for structural change, with calls for antiracist and transformative PH practices centered on and in the pursuit of equity.[3] There has also been increasing and urgent calls for health equity to be more firmly centered in PH education and practice.

Cultural safety is an applied equity concept that has received little attention in the PH field in the United States despite its uptake in other international contexts. "Cultural safety can be viewed on a continuum" that moves from cultural awareness to cultural sensitivity to cultural safety; it "is inherently reflexive as a practice" and requires health care providers to identify and understand their own sets of values and norms while considering how these values and norms might influence how their patients receive health care services.[4(p2)] Indigenous Peoples in the United States may benefit from the operationalizing of cultural safety within PH education and practice as it steers its focus from cultural othering to the clear recognition of the power and privilege of the PH field in relation to tribal communities. PH professionals in the United States, however, require cultural safety frameworks and tools for transformation toward true equity for Indigenous Peoples.

In this article, we propose that such frameworks and tools should not seek to create only awareness of or perceptions of being competent with the cultural norms and practices of marginalized communities. We have seen the harm of falsely embodied cultural competence and exotic othering that occurs within many Indigenous PH spaces, instead of providing PH professionals the resources to look at themselves with the intent to move forward toward true equity.[5] We premise that an internal assessment of dominant cultural beliefs and practices is necessary to create a transformation toward equity.[5]

POSITIONALITY

Because this article discusses cultural safety as it applies to Indigenous Peoples, it is appropriate and expected to provide insight into the contexts and structures influencing the authors.[6] The first author (M. C.) grew up in a White, middle-class, agricultural family within a community of strong Protestant and Catholic traditions and political conservatism. She moved to a metropolitan community in Alaska, where for the first time she lived within a diverse community with a significant Indigenous community presence. The senior author (N. R.) is an enrolled member of the Deninu K'ue First Nation, an Indigenous public health scholar, and former clinician. As authors, we embody within this article the words of renowned Indigenous PH physician and scholar Donald Warne, MD, MPH, who states if "we are ever going to get to equity, we have to walk through truth, even when it's unpleasant. Even when it makes us uncomfortable."[7]

BACKGROUND

Two primary documents, the *10 Essential Public Health Services* and the *Public Health Code of Ethics*, guide PH professional aspirations, key functions, and roles in the United States. Both the *Code of Ethics* and the *10 Essential Services* have recently been revised (in 2019 and 2020, respectively) after extensive input from PH professionals.[3,8] Within the most recent revision to the *10 Essential Services*, which are framed within a circle, a significant edit resulted in the centering of "equity" within the circle (ph.phnci.net/10ephs). The revision also updated language to reflect the embedding of equity into each respective essential service. Additional edits included a call to "correct historical injustices," build a skilled and diverse workforce encompassing "cultural competencies," and place an

AJPH October 2023, Vol 113, No. 10

emphasis on the role of PH in the development or reformation of infrastructures and systems as opposed to the previous focus on innovation and research.[3]

Updates to the *Code of Ethics* also reflect more explicit identification of the need to address health equity, inclusivity, and justice.[8] Although the *Code of Ethics* is not a checklist or rulebook, it does lay out guidance for organizational and individual reflection as well as for the professional development necessary to correct the structural and cultural factors adversely affecting PH services and population health outcomes.[9] The equity calls within the core PH documents echo a national trend to recognize the structural factors, or determinants of health, integral to addressing health inequities within the United States.[1] Other PH-specific literature notes that health inequities can only be corrected by addressing root structural issues underlying population health.[10]

Indigenous Peoples

Indigenous Peoples experience notable health inequities in the United States and associated territories. Globally, Indigenous Peoples are identified as distinct social, cultural, and political groups or nations who were the original residents and stewards within a region long before settler colonization and modern-day political boundaries.[11] For the purposes of this article, "Indigenous Peoples" refers to the original residents of the United States and associated territories, including persons commonly identified as American Indian, Alaska Native, Native Hawaiian, Chamorro, Samoan, or other Pacific Islanders. However, it must be noted that these identifiers (e.g., Pacific Islanders, Alaska Native) were created for the purpose and convenience of racist and colonial policies rather than directed by Indigenous Peoples themselves.[12]

Although distinctive and autonomous, Indigenous Peoples do share overlapping experiences of colonization.[12,13] Colonization refers to the forced process and worldview in which so-called "superior" or "universal" cultural norms, expectations, and teachings are imposed by non-Indigenous settlers to a region.[14] Colonization established—often violently—new conditions for Indigenous Peoples within a White, male, and human supremacy–orientated society, often labeling them either explicitly or implicitly as an inferior or "other" with consequential experiences of genocide, exploitation, racism, and historical trauma.[14]

Colonization's outcomes of genocide, exploitation, racism, and historical trauma have reverberating effects on current-day health inequities for Indigenous Peoples.[14] Compared with non-Hispanic Whites in the United States, Indigenous Peoples have increased rates of chronic conditions, including cancer, diabetes, and heart disease.[2] Indigenous Peoples also have lower educational attainment and are much more likely to be low-income or impoverished.[2] These health inequities are not the result of individual, community, biological, or genetic predispositions but are the direct result of the cumulative impacts of colonization and racism as key determinants of health.[15]

Colonization creates conditions that undermine fundamental determinants of health within Indigenous communities. For instance, the United States has demonstrated historically poor adherence to treaties with Indigenous Peoples, leading to significant gaps and underfunding within educational and health care systems.[2,13] One contributing factor to underfunding can be traced to undercounting within the US Census,[16] which plays an integral role in funding allocation and resource planning. Undercounting of Indigenous Peoples in health monitoring and surveillance systems was powerfully demonstrated during the COVID-19 pandemic.[17] Indigenous Peoples' case counts and mortality reports were underreported because of arbitrary aggregation thresholds requiring grassroots efforts to identify and track case and mortality inequities to ensure equitable distribution of vaccines.[17]

There are additional policy factors contributing to the data obfuscation of Indigenous Peoples beyond the Census, including those facilitating diaspora. Many Indigenous Peoples have been forcibly removed from their traditional homelands, with later relocation to urban centers,[18] or have had other treaty rights allowing relocation for educational or economic purposes.[13] PH professionals work in communities with Indigenous Peoples and may be unaware that they do so. PH professionals need to be aware not only of the presence and histories of Indigenous Peoples in their communities but also of the systems and power dynamics affecting the Indigenous determinants of health. The existing PH literature and developed interventions often continue to neglect many of the root causes of the determinants of Indigenous Peoples' health (e.g., colonialism as a determinant of health), prioritizing individual or interpersonal interventions rather than addressing the systems creating health inequities.[10]

Cultural Safety

Cultural safety is one applied equity concept that may support the improvement of health outcomes and the relationship between Indigenous Peoples and PH. Cultural safety was originally conceptualized by nurses in response to the inequities experienced by Māori Peoples of Aotearoa (New Zealand) that needed to be addressed by examining the power imbalance between patients and providers.[19] Although there is no singular definition or operationalization of cultural safety,[20] a consistent element that separates cultural safety from cultural competency or humility is the individual and organizational responsibility to recognize and examine the structural relationships of power in every context.[21] Anderson et al.[21] additionally stated that

> [r]ather than focusing on exotic belief systems of people from different ethnocultural backgrounds and treating each group as a distinct entity, we are challenged, instead, to examine the unequal relations of power that are the legacy of the colonial past and neocolonial present.[21(pp196–197)]

The recent increase in cultural safety literature has paralleled the increase in literature on the need to recognize and address biases, prejudice, and racism.[22] Cultural safety, however, has had less traction within the United States compared with the international context to date. There is some speculation that this has roots in the United States' identity as an independent nation rather than a Commonwealth country as well as difficulty in acknowledging existing structures as inequitable.[23]

Cultural safety requires more than acknowledgment of implicit or internalized biases or racism. Cultural safety demands recognition of and action upon the relationships of racism, colonization, and power at the institutional levels of society where immense privileges and power are conferred to the select few.[19,21] Cultural safety shifts the solution of power imbalances and health inequities from Indigenous Peoples to the non-Indigenous culture, as the latter is the main contributor to the problem and therefore is also key to any solutions.[5]

As colonization is the imposition of practices and worldviews creating conditions of superiority or universal cultural norms, decolonization may therefore be described as the process of countering Western-imposed ideals of superiority and homogeneity. Decolonization respects the rights and autonomy of Indigenous Peoples to develop and practice social and organizational structures (i.e., family, health, governance, education) embedded within cultural values as equal to those within Western or European systems of thought and practice.[14] Supporting Indigenous Peoples' decolonization alongside Western-based PH system transformation toward true equity requires ongoing acknowledgment, key actions, and adjustments made to the existing relationships of unbalanced power between Indigenous Nations and the PH profession.

KEY CONCEPTS OF CULTURAL SAFETY

Although cultural safety does not have a universal definition or procedure, several elements are noted consistently within the literature. First, cultural safety is different from cultural competency or humility in its demands to both recognize and transform the existing power relationships within systems. The relationships of power between people and between people and institutions are consistently identified as key components of cultural safety.[20,21,23] Cultural safety goes beyond acknowledging or learning about other cultures, bias, or racism; it requires "personal recognition and then action"[5] upon the imbalances of power that are the foundational root of health inequities. Cultural safety addresses the imbalances of power formed within colonization that are the structural underpinnings of health inequities, particularly for Indigenous Peoples.[20,23] Box 1 provides a summary comparison between key aspects of cultural competency and cultural safety.

Reflexivity is another key element identified within the cultural safety literature.[4,23,24] Reflexivity as both a term and process has long-documented use

BOX 1— Comparison of Key Concepts Between Cultural Safety and Cultural Competency

Cultural Competency	Cultural Safety
• Ethnic or cultural knowledge • Skills and attitudes • Implies achievement • Checking boxes • Implies expertise • Individualized • Indigenous culture holds the solution • Asks: What knowledge do I have?	• Historical contexts • Reflexivity • Process • Power relationships and structures • Decolonization • Systemic and individual • Non-Indigenous culture created the problem and holds the solution • Asks: How was this knowledge produced?

Source. Adapted from information provided by references 5, 19–21, 23, and 24.

AJPH October 2023, Vol 113, No. 10

in qualitative research areas, having a more recent presence in PH and health literature.[24] Reflexivity is the process of recognizing one's position within a system's context and translating that examination into systemic change of norms, values, and structures.[4,25] Reflexivity is an advancement beyond reflection because reflection ultimately focuses on internal, individualistic processes and outcomes rather than systems.[25] Reflexivity also challenges the implied neutrality or objectivity of reflection, as cultural norms and values are neither neutral or apolitical.[24]

Another main element in cultural safety literature is the concept of space. Space has been described as the process of maintaining openings or opportunities for other perspectives, voices, and realities.[21] Leaving space emphasizes a deliberate process of not knowing or not being an expert,[19] which reduces the current privileging of Western (White) ways of knowing and doing. Many PH practitioners are trained in Western-based contexts, and space can open power sharing with those not grounded within Western or formalized academic ways of knowing or doing.[23] Space making removes the demands of expertise and provides the opportunity for PH professionals to be allies and share the work of cultural safety even when they are not Indigenous or another minority person.[5]

Finally, cultural safety is a process. Compared with the implied achievements or expertise within cultural competency, cultural safety has no checklist or arrival.[19] It is instead the ongoing work and commitment of individuals and institutions toward health equity, power sharing, systems change, and decolonization.[19,24] Cultural safety develops from the cumulative impact of numerous small decisions or behaviors rather than a singular event, training, or workshop.[5,22]

THE JOURNEY FORWARD

As noted in the section on "Cultural Safety," the concept of cultural safety is not currently prevalent in US-based resources or literature; however, it seems well-suited for meeting the calls for equity within PH. Although gaps remain in cultural safety interventions and implementation,[20] cultural safety may be the equity framework that best parallels the calls in PH core documents to address population health inequities at their foundational levels.

Cultural safety differs from its two predecessors, cultural competency and cultural humility, in its key themes of power, reflexivity, space, and process.[19,20] Cultural safety places the onus on PH professionals and organizations to transform both themselves and the systems in which they work. PH services must move beyond individual and interpersonal levels and begin to address the structural and systemic foundations of health, particularly for Indigenous Peoples. Cultural safety is an embodied skill that all PH providers need to develop, as Indigenous Peoples live, work, and play in all parts of the United States and are therefore affected by PH policies and practices. PH professionals must be aware of how internal and professional power dynamics influence Indigenous health. Given indications that some PH organizations may be practicing cultural safety without realizing they do so,[23] research about cultural safety understanding and practice in the US context is important. It will also be important to further define and operationalize cultural safety as it applies to Indigenous Peoples themselves as copartners.[20] Evaluation is needed of both the process and the outcomes of how PH transforms individual and organizational practice toward decolonization and equity.

Indigenous health inequities will continue to flourish until PH addresses and corrects the privileged and inequitable systems of power and relationships innate within the field.[10,12] The ability of PH to practice cultural safety requires education, training, and resources to develop the necessary skills to support decolonized systems while also uplifting and acknowledging the inherent strengths within Indigenous Nations. AJPH

CORRESPONDENCE

Correspondence should be sent to Megan Carlson, Department of Population Health, School of Medicine and Health Sciences, University of North Dakota, 1301 N Columbia Rd, Stop 9037, Grand Forks, ND, 58202 (e-mail: megancarlson.ak@gmail.com). Reprints can be ordered at http://www.ajph.org by clicking the "Reprints" link.

PUBLICATION INFORMATION

Full Citation: Carlson M, Redvers N. Indigenous Peoples and cultural safety in public health. *Am J Public Health*. 2023;113(10):1059–1063.

Acceptance Date: June 6, 2023.

DOI: https://doi.org/10.2105/AJPH.2023.307363

CONTRIBUTORS

M. Carlson and N. Redvers performed data curation, wrote the original draft, and reviewed and edited the article. M. Carlson was responsible for conceptualization and methodology.

CONFLICTS OF INTEREST

The authors have no conflicts of interest to declare.

REFERENCES

1. Office of Disease Prevention and Health Promotion. Health Equity and Health Disparities Environmental Scan. 2022. Available at: https://health.gov/sites/default/files/2022-04/HP2030-HealthEquityEnvironmentalScan.pdf. Accessed June 6, 2022.
2. US Commission on Civil Rights. Broken promises: continuing federal funding shortfall for Native Americans. 2018. Available at: https://www.usccr.gov/files/pubs/2018/12-20-Broken-Promises.pdf. Accessed October 4, 2021.

3. Public Health National Center for Innovations. 10 Essential Public Health Services Toolkit. September 2020. Available at: ph.phnci.net/10ephs. Accessed June 7, 2022.
4. Mashford-Pringle A, Tan S, Stutz S, Tjong G. Designing accountability measures for health professionals: results from a community-based micro-credential: case study on Indigenous cultural safety. *BMC Public Health.* 2023;23(1):1–10. https://doi.org/10.1186/s12889-023-15721-9
5. Curtis E. Achieving health equity: cultural competency vs cultural safety? Webinar: The Beryl Institute. June 14, 2022.
6. Lock M, McMillan F, Bennett B, et al. Position statement: research and reconciliation with Indigenous Peoples in rural health journals. *Aust J Rural Health.* 2022;30(1):6–7. https://doi.org/10.1111/ajr.12834
7. Medical News Today. The impact of historical trauma on American Indian health equity. Updated July 11, 2022. Available at: https://www.medicalnewstoday.com/articles/the-impact-of-historical-trauma-on-american-indian-health-equity. Accessed June 7, 2022.
8. American Public Health Association. Public Health Code of Ethics. 2019. Available at: https://www.apha.org/-/media/files/pdf/membergroups/ethics/code_of_ethics.ashx. Accessed May 17, 2022.
9. Lee LM, Ortiz SE, Pavela G, Jennings B. Public Health Code of Ethics: deliberative decision-making and reflective practice. *Am J Public Health.* 2020;110(4):489–491. https://doi.org/10.2105/AJPH.2020.305568
10. Plamondon KM, Bottorff JL, Caxaj CS, Graham ID. The integration of evidence from the Commission on Social Determinants of Health in the field of health equity: a scoping review. *Crit Public Health.* 2020;30(4):415–428. https://doi.org/10.1080/09581596.2018.1551613
11. United Nations Declaration on the Rights of Indigenous Peoples. 2007. Available at: https://www.un.org/development/desa/indigenouspeoples/wp-content/uploads/sites/19/2018/11/UNDRIP_E_web.pdf. Accessed June 7, 2022.
12. Gartner DR, Wilbur RE, McCoy ML. "American Indian" as a racial category in public health: implications for communities and practice. *Am J Public Health.* 2021;111(11):1969–1975. https://doi.org/10.2105/AJPH.2021.306465
13. Morey BN, Tulua A, Tanjasiri SP, et al. Structural racism and its effects on Native Hawaiians and Pacific Islanders in the United States: issues of health equity, census undercounting, and voter disenfranchisement. *AAPI Nexus.* 2020;17(1 & 2):43–76.
14. Redvers N, Yellow Bird M, Quinn D, Yunkaporta T, Arabena K. Molecular decolonization: an Indigenous microcosm perspective of planetary health. *Int J Environ Res Public Health.* 2020;17(12):4586. https://doi.org/10.3390/ijerph17124586
15. Mitchell T. Colonial trauma: complex, continuous, collective, cumulative and compounding effects on the health of Indigenous Peoples in Canada and beyond. *Int J Indig Health.* 2019;14(2):74–94. https://doi.org/10.32799/ijih.v14i2.32251
16. Krieger N. The US Census and the people's health: public health engagement from enslavement and "Indians not taxed" to census tracts and health equity (1790–2018). *Am J Public Health.* 2019;109(8):1092–1100. https://doi.org/10.2105/AJPH.2019.305017
17. Penaia CS, Morey BN, Thomas KB, et al. Disparities in Native Hawaiian and Pacific Islander COVID-19 mortality: a community-driven data response. *Am J Public Health.* 2021;111(suppl 2):S49–S52. https://doi.org/10.2105/AJPH.2021.306370
18. Sheldon BL. Legal and historical roots of health care for American Indians and Alaska Natives in the United States. Kaiser Family Foundation. 2004. Available at: https://www.kff.org/wp-content/uploads/2013/01/legal-and-historical-roots-of-health-care-for-american-indians-and-alaska-natives-in-the-united-states.pdf. Accessed October 24, 2021.
19. Curtis E, Jones R, Tipene-Leach D, et al. Why cultural safety rather than cultural competency is required to achieve health equity: a literature review and recommended definition. *Int J Equity Health.* 2019;18(1):174. https://doi.org/10.1186/s12939-019-1082-3
20. Bowra A, Howard L, Mashford-Pringle A, Ruggiero ED. Indigenous cultural safety training in health, education, and social service work. *Soc Sci Protoc.* 2020;3:1–9. https://doi.org/10.7565/ssp.2020.2815
21. Anderson J, Perry J, Blue C, et al. "Rewriting" cultural safety within the postcolonial and postnational feminist project: toward new epistemologies of healing. *ANS Adv Nurs Sci.* 2003;26(3):196–214. https://doi.org/10.1097/00012272-200307000-00005
22. Croskerry P, Singhal G, Mamede S. Cognitive debiasing 2: impediments to and strategies for change. *BMJ Qual Saf.* 2013;22(suppl 2):ii65–ii72. https://doi.org/10.1136/bmjqs-2012-001713
23. Darroch F, Giles A, Sanderson P, et al. The United States does CAIR about cultural safety: examining cultural safety within Indigenous health contexts in Canada and the United States. *J Transcult Nurs.* 2017;28(3):269–277. https://doi.org/10.1177/1043659616634170
24. Gopal DP, Douglass C, Wong S, Khan I, Lokugamage AU. Reflexivity, cultural safety, and improving the health of racially minoritised communities. *Lancet.* 2022;399(10335):1581–1582. https://doi.org/10.1016/S0140-6736(22)00459-7
25. Liwanag HJ, Rhule E. Dialogical reflexivity towards collective action to transform global health. *BMJ Glob Health.* 2021;6(8):e006825. https://doi.org/10.1136/bmjgh-2021-006825

Teaching Systems Thinking as a Foundational Public Health Competency Can Be Improved

Ligia Paina, PhD, MHS, and Jeffrey Glenn, DrPH, MPA

ABOUT THE AUTHORS

Ligia Paina is with the Department of International Health, Johns Hopkins Bloomberg School of Public Health, Johns Hopkins University, Baltimore, MD. Jeffrey Glenn is with the Department of Public Health, College of Life Sciences, Brigham Young University, Provo, UT.

AJPH October 2023, Vol 113, No. 10

Public health decision-making often deals with problems that do not have a single perfect solution; the solutions' effectiveness depends highly on the context in which they are applied, and they often unfold in uncertain, complex environments. The recent COVID-19 pandemic response provides a perfect example of a "wicked problem."[1–3] At the height of the pandemic, public health professionals had to make decisions without perfect information or sufficient resources, and that at times were at odds with political priorities. Wicked problems like this one are exactly what our graduate education programs should prepare the future public health workforce for.[4–8]

Locally and globally, we have seen increasing calls for problem solving in health to move away from linear thinking and "cookie-cutter" solutions and toward systems thinking and a holistic discourse around identifying and implementing solutions. This approach allows us to better appreciate the richness that arises from the diverse, interrelated, and interdependent components of systems designed to sustain health and well-being.[7,9,10] Systems thinking is defined in varied ways; in practice, its key features involve iterative analysis and problem-solving processes to understand the context, history, and actors related to a particular problem and the pathways through which things influence one another in a whole—a system.[11] Systems thinking can be as much an art as a science and a skill honed though experience over time. The theories, methods, and approaches for systems thinking arise from many disciplines; although many have been applied to public health, the field remains diverse and there are ongoing calls for advancing the application of systems thinking in public health.[11–15] Graduate courses on this topic can help guide those new to the material through this vast territory, and they provide learners with the foundation upon which to apply systems thinking in their future careers.

The calls for advancing systems thinking in public health, however, have not been met with similar efforts to ensure that graduate education programs prepare future public health professionals to apply systems thinking. In fact, the evidence is scarce on how systems thinking should be taught as part of public health and on whether current graduate education programs should prepare graduates to apply systems thinking. Given the urgency to ensure that the public health workforce is prepared to respond to wicked problems, what is graduate public health education currently doing and what else is needed to better prepare future generations of public health systems thinkers?

SYSTEMS THINKING COMPETENCY

The Council on Education for Public Health (CEPH) is an independent agency recognized by the US Department of Education to accredit schools of public health and public health programs outside of schools of public health.[16] The CEPH foundational knowledge areas, learning objectives, and competencies required for accredited public health programs have been a cornerstone advancing the development of a strong public health workforce.[17,18] CEPH requirements, which differ depending on the type of degree (i.e., bachelor's, professional graduate, academic graduate), serve to support the standardization of public health education and raise the bar on how public health is taught across public health programs in the United States. The competencies specific to master of public health (MPH) programs and other professional public health graduate degrees (i.e., some master of science in public health [MSPH] programs) currently recognize the importance of evidence-based approaches, understanding

BOX 1— Council on Education for Public Health (CEPH) Systems Thinking Competency for Master of Public Health (MPH) Programs

2016 Competency description: Apply systems thinking tools to a public health issue
2021 Competency description: Apply a systems thinking tool to visually represent a public health issue in a format other than standard narrative[a]

[a]Systems thinking tools depict or map complex relationships, demonstrating, for example, how component parts of a system interact with and influence one another. Examples include causal loop diagrams, systems archetypes, network analyses, and concept maps. Logic models and evidence tables are not sufficient to address this competency.

public health and health care systems, planning and management to promote health, policy in public health, leadership, communication, interprofessional or intersectoral practice, and systems thinking. However, systems thinking competency was one of the most recently added and has little guidance associated with it.

The CEPH introduced the systems thinking competency in the 2016 revision of its accreditation criteria, as one of its 22 foundational competencies for the MPH and other professional public health graduate degrees. The initial language for this competency (Box 1) referred broadly to the application of systems thinking tools and provided no additional explanation about how graduate programs could implement this competency or assess their courses to demonstrate it was met. The CEPH amended this competency in 2021 to address some of these gaps and specifically require the use of a systems thinking tool to create a visual representation of a public health issue. This revised document also included a short footnote with additional guidance and examples to assist programs in understanding and assessing this competency. A review of how this competency has been implemented to date has not yet been identified in the literature.

SYSTEMS THINKING IN ACCREDITATION APPLICATIONS

To gain a better understanding of how different programs are incorporating systems thinking into their curricula, we accessed the Self-Study and Accreditation Report database on the CEPH Web site[16] and reviewed the self-study applications submitted by all 90 MPH programs that applied for accreditation between 2018 and 2021, using the 2016 criteria that included the new systems thinking competency. Although most MSPH programs are considered academic degree programs, some are considered professional degree programs. Those MSPH programs that are considered professional degree programs are subject to the same CEPH accreditation standards as MPH programs. All 90 of the programs we included in our analysis were MPH programs since none of the professional MSPH programs applied for accreditation during our review period. Although 2018 was the first year in which programs were able to apply using the new (2016) criteria, they were permitted to choose between using the old or new criteria. Nine programs used the new criteria and 18 programs used the old criteria. In total, 108 MPH programs applied for accreditation during our review period. We reviewed only the 90 that applied using the new criteria. After 2018, all programs were required to use the new criteria. At the time of this review, no program had yet applied based on the revised 2021 competency. The CEPH considers programs to be compliant with a competency if they demonstrate that students are both taught a concept and assessed on it, based on supporting documentation such as syllabi and assignment instructions. The percentage of applications assessed by the CEPH as compliant with the systems thinking competency after the initial application submission increased each year during the timeframe of our analysis, from 33% in 2018 to 95% in 2021.

Our analysis resulted in two additional important observations. First, the systems thinking competency is being addressed in many ways across MPH programs. Although only three programs require students to take an entire course dedicated to systems thinking, most programs incorporate this competency into another required public health course. The most common courses in which the systems thinking competency is being covered are leadership and management courses (27/90 programs), environmental health courses (20/90 programs), health policy courses (19/90 programs), and health care systems courses (18/90 programs). However, the other programs addressed systems thinking in a wide variety of other types of courses, including epidemiology (14/90), global health (7/90), and behavioral health (9/90) courses. Many programs (27/90) reported addressing systems thinking in more than one course.

Second, the approaches for teaching systems thinking rely heavily on tools focused on visual representations, many of which specifically mention causal loop diagrams. Based on the applications we reviewed, 46 of the 90 programs assessed the systems thinking competency using a visual aid. Other methods of assessment were also used, the most common being a paper or essay (36/90 programs). This appears to be a main driver of the 2021 competency revision to require the use of a visual aid and provide causal loop diagrams as an illustrative example. Because of the heterogeneity in approaches to integrating systems thinking in the curriculum, it is difficult to tell whether sufficient time is spent on the topic. It is also difficult to determine whether students are introduced to concepts and tools or also have the opportunity to apply them.

FUTURE OPPORTUNITIES

Although systems thinking is listed last among the CEPH MPH foundational competencies, we argue that it should be considered a cross-cutting skill, critical for the achievement of all other competencies. Based on our review of MPH CEPH accreditation applications and our experience teaching future generations of public health professionals to apply systems thinking to their work, we offer the following suggestions:

1. The CEPH should expand the current systems thinking competency to strengthen the connection to the current evidence base and practice for applying systems thinking.
2. The CEPH and public health educators should invest in efforts to generate evidence on ways in which applied systems thinking is benefiting public health initiatives and on how the needed skills can be taught and assessed in a graduate school setting.
3. Educators, practitioners, and the CEPH can do more to promote systems thinking practices and resources and encourage their integration into graduate public health training curricula.

Expand Competency

We applaud the CEPH and all accredited MPH programs for prioritizing systems thinking and moving the field forward by establishing the systems thinking competency, but the overemphasis on visual aids in an attempt to standardize the assessment is a reductionist approach that is contrary to the core idea of systems thinking as a lens that helps public health professionals address complexity. We see the cross-cutting systems thinking competency as unique among the MPH competencies in that it does not always lend itself to operationalization and assessment in the same way as the others. An expanded systems thinking competency could shift the emphasis away from tools and approaches to map and understand complex systems to strategies used to manage complexity, make decisions under uncertain conditions, and influence system transformation. A single course or lecture may not single-handedly satisfy an expanded requirement. Rather than meeting the criteria by demonstrating how systems thinking is assessed in at least one course (as is done with the other competencies), the CEPH could encourage or even require programs to explain how systems thinking (beyond just visual aids) is integrated at multiple points within a curriculum.

Generate Evidence

Given the variety of ways in which systems thinking is taught and assessed, it is unclear whether the systems thinking competency fully captures learners' readiness and confidence to apply a systems approach to solving complex problems in their future public health endeavors. Employers can be tapped to help inform what systems thinking skills are specifically in demand given the current public health climate and postpandemic recovery efforts in particular.

Promote Practices and Resources

Although the introduction of a CEPH competency on systems thinking is an important step in advancing its use in public health among the next generation of practitioners, we observe an opportunity to leverage learning from one another to the benefit of advancing public health education. Illustrative, not comprehensive, actions that educators, practitioners, and public health professional organizations could take include the following:

- Create linkages with broader communities who have taught systems thinking in practice in other contexts (e.g., systems engineering, systems thinking in practice [or STIP] programs at Open University).
- Engage in monitoring and learning from experiences by linking with the American Public Health Association and others to highlight systems thinking at mainstream public health conferences and events.
- Strengthen ties between academia and practice through adaptation of systems thinking curricula beyond

schools and programs of public health into training for the public health workforce.
- Create a repository of teaching systems thinking resources (e.g., learning objectives associated with systems thinking classes and assignments, teaching cases, and strategies for facilitating systems thinking), ideally linked to an existing repository with teaching resources for public health, such as the one hosted by the Association of Schools and Programs of Public Health.[19]

The potential value of systems thinking will not be realized until its use becomes normalized across the field. Identifying and sharing good practices in teaching systems thinking, including ways for teachers and nonteachers of systems thinking to connect with and expand their own teaching portfolio beyond a basic tool set, is a good place to start. More research beyond our brief review is needed into the way systems thinking is taught and assessed in US-based graduate public health programs. Additional opportunities involve learning about how other disciplines and non-US universities approach this topic. AJPH

CORRESPONDENCE

Correspondence should be sent to Jeffrey Glenn, 2032 LSB, Provo, UT 84602 (e-mail: jeff_glenn@byu.edu). Reprints can be ordered at http://www.ajph.org by clicking the "Reprints" link.

PUBLICATION INFORMATION

Full Citation: Paina L, Glenn J. Teaching systems thinking as a foundational public health competency can be improved. *Am J Public Health*. 2023;113(10):1064–1067.

Acceptance Date: June 14, 2023.

DOI: https://doi.org/10.2105/AJPH.2023.307368

CONTRIBUTORS

Both authors contributed equally to this article.

CONFLICTS OF INTEREST

The authors declare no conflicts of interest.

REFERENCES

1. Auld G, Bernstein S, Cashore B, Levin K. Managing pandemics as super wicked problems: lessons from, and for, COVID-19 and the climate crisis. *Policy Sci.* 2021;54(4):707–728. https://doi.org/10.1007/s11077-021-09442-2
2. Rittel HWJ, Webber MM. Dilemmas in a general theory of planning. *Policy Sci.* 1973;4(2):155–169. https://doi.org/10.1007/BF01405730
3. Haley D, Paucar-Caceres A, Schlindwein S. A critical inquiry into the value of systems thinking in the time of COVID-19 crisis. *Systems.* 2021;9(1):13. https://doi.org/10.3390/systems9010013
4. Frenk J, Chen L, Bhutta ZA, et al. Health professionals for a new century: transforming education to strengthen health systems in an interdependent world. *Educación Médica.* 2015;16(1)9–16. https://doi.org/10.1016/j.edumed.2015.04.011
5. Frenk J, Chen LC, Chandran L, et al. Challenges and opportunities for educating health professionals after the COVID-19 pandemic. *Lancet.* 2022;400(10362):1539–1556. https://doi.org/10.1016/S0140-6736(22)02092-X
6. Shen AK. Finding a way to address a wicked problem: vaccines, vaccination, and a shared understanding. *Hum Vaccin Immunother.* 2020;16(5):1030–1033. https://doi.org/10.1080/21645515.2019.1695458
7. Leischow SJ, Best A, Trochim WM, et al. Systems thinking to improve the public's health. *Am J Prev Med.* 2008;35(2 suppl):S196–S203. https://doi.org/10.1016/j.amepre.2008.05.014
8. Trochim WM, Cabrera DA, Milstein B, Gallagher RS, Leischow SJ. Practical challenges of systems thinking and modeling in public health. *Am J Public Health.* 2006;96(3):538–546. https://doi.org/10.2105/AJPH.2005.066001
9. Russell E, Swanson RC, Atun R, Nishtar S, Chunharas S. Systems thinking for the post-2015 agenda. *Lancet.* 2014;383(9935):2124–2125. https://doi.org/10.1016/S0140-6736(14)61028-X
10. Adam T, De Savigny D. Systems thinking for strengthening health systems in LMICs: need for a paradigm shift. *Health Policy Plan.* 2012;27(suppl 4):iv1–iv3. https://doi.org/10.1093/heapol/czs084
11. Peters DH. The application of systems thinking in health: why use systems thinking? *Health Res Policy Sys.* 2014;12(1):51. https://doi.org/10.1186/1478-4505-12-51
12. Paina L, Bennett S, Ssengooba F, Peters DH. Advancing the application of systems thinking in health: exploring dual practice and its management in Kampala, Uganda. *Health Res Policy Syst.* 2014;12(1):41. https://doi.org/10.1186/1478-4505-12-41
13. Glenn J, Kamara K, Umar ZA, Chahine T, Daulaire N, Bossert T. Applied systems thinking: a viable approach to identify leverage points for accelerating progress towards ending neglected tropical diseases. *Health Res Policy Syst.* 2020;18(1):56. https://doi.org/10.1186/s12961-020-00570-4
14. Thelen J, Sant Fruchtman C, Bilal M, et al. Development of the Systems Thinking for Health Actions framework: a literature review and a case study. *BMJ Glob Health.* 2023;8(3):e010191. https://doi.org/10.1136/bmjgh-2022-010191
15. Chughtai S, Blanchet K. Systems thinking in public health: a bibliographic contribution to a meta-narrative review. *Health Policy Plan.* 2017:32(4):585–594. https://doi.org/10.1093/heapol/czw159
16. Council on Education for Public Health. Available at: https://ceph.org. Accessed May 4, 2023.
17. Jacobsen KH, Zeraye HA, Bisesi MS, Gartin M, Malouin RA, Waggett CE. Master of public health global health concentration competencies: preparing culturally skilled practitioners to serve internationally, nationally, and locally. *Am J Public Health.* 2019;109(9):1189–1190. https://doi.org/10.2105/AJPH.2019.305208
18. Park C, Migliaccio G, Edberg M, Frehywot S, Johnson G. Analysis of CEPH-accredited DrPH programs in the United States: a mixed-methods study. *PLoS One.* 2021;16(2):e0245892. https://doi.org/10.1371/journal.pone.0245892
19. Association of Schools and Programs of Public Health (ASPPH). Education. Available at: https://aspph.org/education-practice-research/education. Accessed June 8, 2023.

The Abortion Double Bind

Dov Fox, JD, DPhil, LLM

ABOUT THE AUTHOR

Dov Fox is the Herzog Research Professor of Law and the director of the Center for Health Law Policy & Bioethics, University of San Diego School of Law, San Diego, CA.

In March 2023, patients and doctors sued Texas for criminalizing abortion care in the face of catastrophic health risks associated with continued pregnancy. Lead plaintiff Amanda Zurawski suffered a dangerous complication at 18 weeks' gestation—preterm premature rupture of membranes—that left no chance her baby could be born alive. But fetal cardiac activity could still be detected, so physicians were legally forbidden from safely ending her pregnancy, or at least they had plausible reason to think that providing Zurawski with an abortion could subject them to felony prosecution. That delayed medical intervention to the point that she became septic and nearly died. The lawsuit asks state courts to make clear that the Texas ban on abortion makes space for clinicians to end a pregnancy when doing so is medically necessary.[1]

Texas does not defend its prohibition by claiming that every such abortion is unlawful. Instead, it says that there is no need to clarify a ban whose medical exceptions already authorize clinicians to end a pregnancy if doing so is necessary to save a patient's life. For all that they disagree about, both sides see eye to eye on the question at issue: whether and when the state's ban allows abortion to avoid serious injury or death. But neither considers a related question that has gotten short shrift in larger debates about abortion since the Supreme Court overruled *Roe v Wade* (*Roe*) last summer in *Dobbs v Jackson Women's Health Organization* (*Dobbs*).

This neglected question goes beyond the rare conditions under which abortion restrictions would still allow clinicians to provide one. Namely, do other parts of the legal system actually demand abortion to save a patient's life or preserve her health? The answer is sometimes yes: that is, when the very procedure that a state bans as first-degree homicide is nevertheless mandated by other laws governing medical practice as essential care. This leaves clinicians in a precarious double bind: trapped between (1) the risk of criminal conviction for ending a pregnancy that is not perilous enough to qualify for the medical exceptions to state abortion bans, and (2) the risk of civil liability for not ending a pregnancy that is too dangerous under either state malpractice law or a federal statute that requires emergency medical treatment.[2]

BETWEEN FELONY AND NEGLIGENCE

There is historical precedent for a modified version of the double bind. It is not about failing to end a pregnancy when that is medically necessary but rather about performing an abortion in a way that is negligent. Before *Roe* was decided, roughly half of the courts that faced this question answered that, yes, malpractice lawsuits could proceed against anyone who harmed a pregnant person by botching the criminalized abortions that the woman herself had sought out. These cases cast her as the victim of misconduct and not as an accomplice who should be barred from recovery for having taken part in criminal activity gone awry. Criminal abortion lawsuits for negligence and wrongful death were permitted not only against back-alley quacks or well-meaning nonprofessionals. They were also allowed against licensed doctors in good standing. What is more, the plaintiff who could show she had been hurt by a badly performed abortion usually won. And so most of these cases awarded damages to injured women or their families if they were killed.[3]

But the double bind is not the same today. For one thing, during the 1950s and 1960s, tort reform did not yet significantly constrain liability and damages for medical malpractice. Since *Roe* was decided, malpractice threats have diminished, and criminal threats have intensified. Moreover, abortion suits for malpractice after the *Dobbs* decision will take on a different form. In the pre-*Roe* era, claims were for the negligent commission of medically unnecessary abortions that clearly violated criminal bans. The fact patterns involved slipshod procedures.

Today's negligence claims will instead be for the omission of medically necessary abortions that wary clinicians had delayed or denied precisely to avoid committing what they believed would be a crime. It is now the difference between a wrongful act and an omission or between wrongful doing and allowing. This distinction looms large in many areas of social and legal life, but it carries less purchase in the context of medicine, where clinicians routinely have not just negative duties (to avoid

AJPH October 2023, Vol 113, No. 10

harming patients by undertaking misadvised interventions) but also affirmative duties (to prevent undue harm from befalling patients by failing to provide beneficial care).[4]

Health care professionals are stuck between the conflicting imperatives of abortion bans and potential civil malpractice suits. They are not setting out to defy the law or act with indifference to patient welfare. They are simply trying to follow confusing and conflicting rules while keeping those under their care safe. They might be able to expect enough sympathy from those who could sue or prosecute them. Perhaps injured patients and their families would not bring a lawsuit for failure to provide a medically necessary abortion if they appreciated that doctors felt their hands were tied. And even district attorneys who want to go after a doctor for performing a medical abortion might pass on trying a case that they are not confident of winning by convincing a jury to convict.

But maybe not.

Meanwhile, for the clinician who is stuck in the middle, the outcome of any such lawsuit or prosecution would be uncertain. What clinician wants to take that risk and be forced to justify their conduct in a trial proceeding? One with a high profile and higher stakes, especially against any criminal charges? Guessing wrong could not only invite harassment and even threats but could also lead to revocation of their medical license or land them in prison. Attorneys' fees alone could be daunting for many practitioners in abortion-restrictive states who are faced with the prospect of terminating a patient's pregnancy to preserve her health or potentially save her life. Malpractice insurance usually does not cover the cost of criminal defense.

BETWEEN FEDERAL AND STATE LAWS

It is not just individual doctors and nurses who might face competing legal obligations in medical emergencies during pregnancy now that *Roe* is gone. Health care institutions could too under a 1986 federal law, the Emergency Medical Treatment and Labor Act (EMTALA). EMTALA requires hospital emergency departments and staff to stabilize any patient in active labor or whose symptoms are so acute that "the absence of immediate medical attention could reasonably be expected" to place that person's health "in serious jeopardy."[5]

Hospitals that violate EMTALA—for example, by turning away an unstable patient who cannot afford care—risk losing their Medicare funding, which can put them out of business. Although EMTALA provides injured patients and their families a private right of action to sue institutions themselves, it is mostly up to the US Department of Health and Human Services (HHS) to implement statutory penalties. So when it comes to the emergency denial of politically contested care such as abortion, EMTALA violations are more likely to be enforced if HHS leadership is under the direction of a presidential administration that supports abortion access.

Indeed, in July 2022, President Biden's HHS clarified that EMTALA's treatment mandate includes ending a dangerous pregnancy, even in states that ban abortion.[6] The HHS guidance includes a nonexhaustive list of emergent conditions in pregnant patients—ultimately leaving it up to the judgment of clinicians to determine whether "the absence of immediate medical attention could reasonably be expected" to place a person's health "in serious jeopardy." The Constitution's Supremacy Clause says that when two laws—one of them federal, the other state—pull citizens in opposite directions, the federal law governs. Accordingly, EMTALA would seem to resolve the abortion double bind in hospital emergency departments because states cannot bar clinicians from providing the emergency abortion care that the federal government commands them to provide.

That is why a federal court enjoined Idaho's ban on providing abortion to the extent that its medical exceptions are less generous than "EMTALA-mandated care."[7] And in May 2023, HHS secretary Xavier Becerra announced active investigations into two hospitals for failing to provide the stabilizing abortion care EMTALA requires. Even so, uncertainty remains in other abortion-restrictive states about whether it is permissible to provide emergency abortion care. And Becerra's statement noted that the HHS lacks such enforcement power for now in Texas.[8]

A federal court there, faced with a similar case, suspended not the abortion ban but the HHS guidance instead, reasoning that EMTALA "is silent as to abortion" and "protects both mothers and unborn children."[9] Texas argued that EMTALA does not supersede or preempt states' power to regulate or prohibit abortion because, however dangerous it would be to continue a patient's pregnancy, ending it would not preserve the life or health of the unborn child, who is also a patient.[10] That Texas ruling has since been appealed to a higher court.

AMBIGUOUS MEDICAL EXEMPTIONS

No matter the state, EMTALA applies only to emergency department care, so practitioners who provide an abortion in other clinical settings must rely on the medical exemptions in their state's ban. These carveouts use phrases such as "serious health risk" and "life-threatening impairment" of a "major bodily function," without narrowing down how bad, how likely, or how imminent a harm must be to qualify.

What if a delay in abortion care causes an unavoidable hysterectomy? How about cancer treatment that is not compatible with pregnancy? This point was also made in the *Dobbs* case by the dissenting justices of the US Supreme Court, who would have affirmed the constitutional right to abortion under *Roe*. They put the challenge like this: "Suppose a patient with pulmonary hypertension has a 30-to-50 percent risk of dying with ongoing pregnancy."[11] Is that enough? As Box 1 shows, these laws do not say.

DELAYED CARE AND ARBITRARY PROSECUTION

Uncertain statutory language pervades medical exemptions, leaving clinicians fearful that providing standard of care abortions they see as clearly health or life preserving might look criminal to an uncompromising prosecutor. No wonder that abortion-restrictive states report vanishingly few abortions being performed under these exceptions—far fewer, the early evidence suggests, than the number required to keep medical crises during pregnancy from getting worse.[12]

Nine months before *Dobbs* overturned *Roe*, Texas first banned abortion in a civil law known as SB 8, the Texas Heartbeat Act. The law authorizes a private citizen to sue anyone else at all for $10 000 in damage awards if it is found that the other person either provided an abortion after about six weeks or facilitated one, for example, by counseling a pregnant person, funding her abortion, or even giving her a ride to the clinic.[13]

When SB 8 went into effect in September 2021, researchers began studying women with pregnancy complications at two Dallas, Texas, hospitals. The researchers found that, with SB 8 looming in the background, twice as many women ended up in the intensive care unit for avoidable life-threatening emergencies than would have before the ban. These are emergencies that could have been prevented if the patients had not been made to wait an average of nine extra days for their conditions to deteriorate.[14]

Medical exceptions to state bans on providing abortion were common before *Roe* was decided too, as was confusion about when and how those exceptions applied. In fact, the Supreme

BOX 1— Representative Medical Exceptions From State Bans on Providing Abortion

State	Statutory Language
Arkansas, Idaho, Mississippi, Oklahoma, South Dakota, and Wisconsin	Providing abortion is a crime unless "necessary" to "preserve the life" or "prevent the death" of a pregnant patient. No exception to preserve health.
Alabama code § 26–23H-3/4	Providing abortion is a crime unless "necessary" to "avert death" or "serious risk of substantial physical impairment of a major bodily function."
Kentucky revised statutes § 311.772	Providing abortion is a crime unless "necessary . . . to prevent the serious, permanent impairment of a life-sustaining organ of a pregnant woman."
Louisiana revised statutes § 40:1061 and 14:87.1	Providing abortion is a crime unless "necessary . . . to prevent the serious, permanent impairment of a life-sustaining organ of a pregnant woman."
Missouri revised statutes § 188.015 and 188.017	Providing abortion is a crime unless the defendant proves "by a preponderance of the evidence" that abortion was necessary "to avert the death of the pregnant woman or for which a delay will create a serious risk of substantial and irreversible physical impairment of a major bodily function."
Tennessee code § 39–15-213	Providing abortion is a crime unless the defendant proves "by a preponderance of the evidence," "based upon the facts known to the physician at the time, that the abortion was necessary to prevent the death of the pregnant woman or to prevent serious risk of substantial and irreversible impairment of a major bodily function."
Texas health & safety code § 170A.002(b)/001(4)	Providing abortion is allowed only if "the pregnant female . . . has a life-threatening physical condition aggravated by, caused by, or arising from a pregnancy that places the female at risk of death or poses a serious risk of substantial impairment of a major bodily function unless the abortion is performed or induced."
West Virginia code § 16–2R-2/-4	"An abortion may not be performed" unless necessary "to avert serious risk of the patient's death or . . . substantial life-threatening physical impairment of a major bodily function, not including psychological or emotional conditions."

Court's first draft of that landmark decision offered a different justification for striking down Texas's ban on all but lifesaving abortions—not for violating a constitutional right of privacy but because the statute was "void for vagueness."[15] That alternative opinion would have invalidated the state's bar on nonemergency abortions on the ground that it gave clinicians insufficient guidance and an unfair lack of notice about what conduct is criminal, inviting arbitrary enforcement through selective prosecution. Obstetricians and gynecologists voice similar concerns about today's medical exemptions.

THE PROBLEM WITH ENUMERATION

Medically needed abortion care is being delayed and denied because doctors are understandably anxious not to cross the line drawn by vague medical exceptions. But that does not mean it would be better for states to specify eligible conditions. Detailed lists might reassure tentative physicians that they would not be prosecuted for performing an abortion in particular circumstances. Yet such preclearance would also operate to suppress the case-by-case discretion that is appropriately responsive to medical context under time-sensitive conditions.[16]

It is precisely that open-ended statutory language about qualifying harms and risks that enables the crucial exercise of reasonable judgment and good faith professionalism—at any rate, for clinicians who are not psychiatrists. That is because most abortion bans limit medical exceptions to physical harms and explicitly exclude psychological and emotional conditions. Accordingly, diagnoses of a woman's depression or suicidality, however real and acute, would not make it legal to provide her with an abortion. Before *Roe* was decided, so-called psychiatric abortions were often deemed too vulnerable to subjectivity or pretext to justify ending unwanted pregnancies by people healthy enough to carry them to term.[17] Yet preserving this measure of clinical discretion is critical for preserving the individualized care that ordinarily resists straightforward preclassification into neatly defined categories.

But the ambiguity of medical exemptions is not the real problem with the abortion double bind. After all, one way out of that bind would be to legislate that clinicians cannot be sued for denying an emergency abortion. Thirty-three states already have far-reaching conscience clauses on the books that shield foreseeably harmful denials of abortion care by clinicians who invoke deeply held moral beliefs. These laws immunize conscientious refusers from being fired, disciplined, or held liable.[18] States could simply expand such liability shields to any withholding of abortion care, whether in the name of conscience or not. But this move would have a pernicious effect: to insulate clinicians from even modest consequences for hurting patients in foreseeable and serious ways that ordinarily amount to malpractice, patient abandonment, or wrongful death.

This points to what is actually a deeper conflict between, on the one hand, the professional obligations that animate those civil and statutory actions and, on the other, the crushing penalties set forth by modern bans that make abortion a crime. Again, the past is instructive. Before *Roe* was decided, police suspicion was rarely triggered by the criminal abortions that licensed clinicians performed safely. It helped that the majority of doctors back then practiced in the privacy of small mom-and-pop shops where no one would tell on them. Others received approval from "abortion committees." These committees operated in many private hospitals that served predominantly White patients who had insurance, thereby excluding many poor people in rural regions or marginalized communities.[19]

Under any medical setting, the legal peril today is more acute. In the pre-*Roe* era, abortions were simple misdemeanors. After *Dobbs*, criminal abortions are high-order felonies. And they are less likely to go under the radar today. A massive reorganization of health care in recent decades has left most doctors practicing in large institutions, where a team of co-workers look over their shoulders. Abortion bans are also enforced through electronic surveillance and bounty-style regimes that solicit informants to sue for a reward.

FROM ASPIRATIONAL TO OPERATIONAL

Clinicians and the groups that represent them should take action both now and in the long term. First, there are ways for clinicians to reduce the legal risks of providing abortions under the discretion that EMTALA and medical exceptions afford them. They can seek free guidance about state law and specific counsel about particular facts, as well as legal representation if they end up being prosecuted for the reasonable exercise of clinical judgment to provide a life- or health-preserving abortion.

Resources at their disposal include the American Medical Association's legal defense fund, public interest coalitions such as the Abortion Defense Network, and private associations such as the Legal Alliance for Reproductive

Rights—even if hospital lawyers and risk managers are presumed to care about institutional liability risks too much to be trusted to reasonably weigh those risks against the medical and professional interests of patients and providers. Guidance on practice standards is also on offer from state medical boards and national organizations such as the American College of Obstetricians and Gynecologists and the Society for Maternal–Fetal Medicine.[20]

LOBBYING FOR LEGISLATIVE REFORM

These medical groups should vigorously lobby legislatures to change bad laws. Beyond outright repeal of abortion bans, there are incremental reforms worth advocating. First is the addition of health-based exceptions to the abortion statutes in such states as Arkansas, Idaho, Mississippi, Oklahoma, South Dakota, and Wisconsin, whose exemptions are limited to saving a life. Second, in Missouri and Tennessee, doctors and nurses can be prosecuted for providing an abortion even if it clearly qualifies for medical exemption. There, groups should press for amendments that shift the burden of proof back to states to prove a clinician has actually violated the criminal law before hauling her into court.

JUDICIAL DEFENSE TO PRACTICE MEDICINE

A final proposal is for state judges. They enjoy a measure of authority to mitigate criminal penalties by establishing justifications or excuses. Even if a prosecutor secured a conviction, judges could reduce the punishment based, for example, on a clinician's reasonable reliance on medical exemptions or good faith effort to heal patients and promote their health. A New Jersey court recognized these reasons in another context, referring to a clinician's charge to put patients first as a "clear mandate of public policy" that "deserves judicial protection" because "the ethical goals of professional conduct are of inestimable social value."[21]

It has been more than a century since courts last flexed their common-law muscles to fashion new affirmative defenses such as duress, entrapment, insanity, necessity, and self-defense. There is reason to recover that muscle memory today when the relationship between the practice of medicine and the rule of law has never felt so fragile. A common-law defense to criminal prosecution would vindicate the reasonable exercise of clinical discretion to respond to patient needs in the ways that medical exemptions and federal statutes like EMTALA were designed to authorize.[22]

CONCLUSIONS

The abortion double bind is untenable. Doctors and nurses who practice medicine in good faith must not be trapped between criminal and civil law or state and federal law. Nor should fear of prosecution undermine professional obligations to exercise reasonable clinical judgment, lest the provision of emergent abortion care continue to be dangerously chilled. Although medical organizations urge critical legislative reforms, cost-free representation and guidance is available to help clinicians navigate these challenges for the sake of patients in need. AJPH

CORRESPONDENCE

Correspondence should be sent to Dov Fox, 5998 Alcala Park, San Diego, CA 92110 (e-mail: dovfox@sandiego.edu). Reprints can be ordered at http://www.ajph.org by clicking the "Reprints" link.

PUBLICATION INFORMATION

Full Citation: Fox D. The abortion double bind. *Am J Public Health*. 2023;113(10):1068–1073.

Acceptance Date: June 15, 2023.

DOI: https://doi.org/10.2105/AJPH.2023.307369

ACKNOWLEDGMENTS

For valuable criticisms and insightful recommendations, the author owes a debt of gratitude to anonymous editors and reviewers for *AJPH* as well as to Liz Parker, publication services librarian at the University of San Diego Legal Research Center.

CONFLICTS OF INTEREST

The author has no conflicts of interest to declare.

REFERENCES

1. *Zurawski v Texas*, No. D-1-GN-23_000968 (Dist. Ct. Travis County March 6, 2023). Available at: https://reproductiverights.org/wp-content/uploads/2023/03/Zurawski-v-State-of-Texas-Complaint.pdf. Accessed June 26, 2023.
2. Mello MM. Resuscitating abortion rights in emergency care. *JAMA Health Forum*. 2022;3(9):e223781. https://doi.org/10.1001/jamahealthforum.2022.3781
3. Reagan L. Victim or accomplice? Crime, medical malpractice, and the construction of the aborting woman in American case law, 1860s–1970. *Columbia J Gend Law*. 2001;10(2):311–332. https://doi.org/10.7916/cjgl.v10i2.2433
4. Centers for Disease Control and Prevention. Four in 5 pregnancy-related deaths in the US are preventable. September 19, 2022. Available at: https://www.cdc.gov/media/releases/2022/p0919-pregnancy-related-deaths.html. Accessed February 21, 2023.
5. Emergency Medical Treatment and Labor Act, 42 U.S.C. § 1395dd.
6. Centers for Medicare & Medicaid Services. Reinforcement of EMTALA obligations specific to patients who are pregnant or are experiencing pregnancy loss. August 25, 2022. Available at: https://www.cms.gov/files/document/qso-22-22-hospitals.pdf. Accessed May 1, 2023.
7. *US v Idaho*, No. 1:22-cv-00329 (D. Idaho February 3, 2023). Available at: https://casetext.com/case/united-states-v-state-2011. Accessed June 26, 2023.
8. Department of Health and Human Services. HHS secretary Xavier Becerra statement on EMTALA enforcement. May 1, 2023. Available at: https://www.hhs.gov/about/news/2023/05/01/hhs-secretary-xavier-becerra-statement-on-emtala-enforcement.html. Accessed June 26, 2023.
9. *State of Texas v Becerra et al.*, No. 5:2022cv00185, document 73 (N.D. Tex. 2022). Available at: https://law.justia.com/cases/federal/district-courts/texas/txndce/5:2022cv00185/365015/73. Accessed June 26, 2023.
10. *State of Texas v Xavier Becerra*, No. 5:22-cv-185-H, document 1 (N.D. Tex. 2022). Available at: https://www.texasattorneygeneral.gov/sites/default/files/

images/executive-management/20220714_1-0_Original%20Complaint%20Biden%20Admin.pdf. Accessed June 26, 2023.

11. *Dobbs et al. v Jackson Women's Health Organization*. (October 2021). Available at: https://www.supremecourt.gov/opinions/21pdf/19-1392_6j37.pdf. Accessed June 26, 2023.
12. Walker AS. Most abortion bans include exceptions. In practice, few are granted. *New York Times*. January 23, 2023. Available at: https://www.nytimes.com/interactive/2023/01/21/us/abortion-ban-exceptions.html. Accessed February 21, 2023.
13. Tex. Health & Safety Code Ann. § 171.208(a)(2). (West 2021). Available at: https://statutes.capitol.texas.gov/Docs/HS/htm/HS.171.htm. Accessed June 26, 2023.
14. Nambiar A, Patel S, Santiago-Munoz P, et al. Maternal morbidity and fetal outcomes among pregnant women at 22 weeks' gestation or less with complications in 2 Texas hospitals after legislation on abortion. *Am J Obstet Gynecol.* 2022; 227(4):648–650.e1. https://doi.org/10.1016/j.ajog.2022.06.060
15. Greenhouse LJ. *Becoming Justice Blackmun: Harry Blackmun's Supreme Court Journey*. New York, NY: Times Books; 2015.
16. Grossman D, Joffe C, Kaller S, et al. Care post-*Roe*: documenting cases of poor-quality care since the *Dobbs* decision. May 2023. Available at: https://www.ansirh.org/sites/default/files/2023-05/Care%20Post-Roe%20Preliminary%20Findings.pdf. Accessed June 28, 2023.
17. Schwartz RA. Abortion on request: the psychiatric implications. *Case West. Reserve Law Rev.* 1972;23(4):840–873. Available at: https://scholarlycommons.law.case.edu/cgi/viewcontent.cgi?article=2902&context=caselrev. Accessed June 26, 2023.
18. Sawicki NN. The conscience defense to malpractice. *Calif Law Rev.* 2020;108:1255–1316. Available at: https://lawecommons.luc.edu/cgi/viewcontent.cgi?article=1680&context=facpubs. Accessed June 26, 2023.
19. Howard H. Therapeutic abortion: ten years' experience with hospital committee control. *Am J Obstet Gynecol.* 1964;89(3):349–355. https://doi.org/10.1016/0002-9378(64)90690-8
20. Watson K. Dark-alley ethics—how to interpret medical exceptions to bans on abortion provision. *N Engl J Med.* 2023;388(13):1240–1245. https://doi.org/10.1056/NEJMms2216234
21. *Pierce v Ortho Pharm. Corp.* N.J. 417, 515 & 521 (Supreme Court of New Jersey 1980). Available at: https://law.justia.com/cases/new-jersey/supreme-court/1980/84-n-j-58-0.html. Accessed June 26, 2023.
22. Fox D. Medical disobedience. *Harv Law Rev.* 2023;136:1030–1111. https://harvardlawreview.org/2023/02/medical-disobedience. Accessed June 26, 2023.

Unpacking Cochrane's Update on Masks and COVID-19

Brian M. Gurbaxani, PhD, Andrew N. Hill, PhD, and Pragna Patel, MD, MPH

ABOUT THE AUTHORS

Brian M. Gurbaxani and Pragna Patel are with the National Center for Immunization and Respiratory Diseases, Centers for Disease Control and Prevention (CDC), Atlanta, GA. Brian M. Gurbaxani is also with the Departments of Electrical and Computer Engineering and Industrial and Systems Engineering, Georgia Institute of Technology, Atlanta. Andrew N. Hill is with the Global Health Center, Division of Parasitic Diseases and Malaria, CDC, and the Department of Biostatistics and Bioinformatics Department, Rollins School of Public Health, Emory University, Atlanta, GA. Pragna Patel is also with the Department of Medicine, Emory University.

AJPH October 2023, Vol 113, No. 10

Recently, the Cochrane Library released its anticipated update on physical interventions to control the spread of respiratory viruses, including masks to contain the spread of severe acute respiratory syndrome coronavirus 2 (SARS-CoV-2).[1] The update was widely read and cited, becoming a point of controversy in the public debate about the efficacy of face masks, as it appeared to contradict both public health guidance[2] and research.[3] The appearance of controversy was in part owing to the methodological approach of Cochrane reviews, which allows inclusion of only randomized controlled trials (RCTs).

The authors added 11 new RCTs and cluster RCTs, of which six were conducted during the COVID-19 pandemic and evaluated various interventions for hygiene, including face masks and hand washing. Only two of the six studies compared use of face masks with no use of masks: one from Denmark, the DANMASK-19 RCT,[4] and one from Bangladesh.[5] But even with these limited, additional data, the appearance of disagreement between the Cochrane review results and public health guidance disappears if infectious disease models are applied, because the models calibrate quite well to the new Cochrane data and, when extrapolated, show that masks can reduce respiratory infections significantly.

TWO NEW COCHRANE REVIEW STUDIES

The DANMASK-19 study had several flaws: it was underpowered; was not able to evaluate the impact of masks as source control (i.e., filtering viral particles directly from the source, the infected wearer); used SARS-CoV-2 antibody testing to detect infection instead of antigen testing, which is used to identify acute illness (so that infection could have happened at any time in the past, not necessarily during the study period); and was conducted at a time of low SARS-CoV-2 circulation.[6,7]

The cluster RCT in Bangladesh was a large study, with more than 340 000 participants, that demonstrated that villages receiving the intervention had increased mask use.[5] Although the study was not designed to demonstrate mask efficacy in reducing infections, it found that increases in mask use correlated with lower SARS-CoV-2 seroprevalence. Because evidence is weighted by the number of participants, the most heavily weighted data for face masks during the COVID-19 pandemic come from the RCT conducted in Bangladesh, representing more than 95% of the new data related to the pandemic that was used in the Cochrane update.

The Cochrane review mentioned many of its own limitations and weaknesses, particularly with regard to face masks and its limited number of robust studies; it, therefore, cautioned against drawing any strong conclusions. Given the strong opinions expressed about the study, Cochrane further clarified that their review should not be used as evidence against mask efficacy per se, noting that the data were not definitive and that masks might be effective at preventing respiratory virus infection.[8]

MASKS AND MATERIALS ENGINEERING

From the standpoint of workplace safety and materials engineers, the debate on masks is something of an enigma: the utility of wearing masks should be obvious. Viruses like SARS-CoV-2 populate the respiratory tract.[9] During talking, singing, coughing, and sneezing, viruses are expelled into the ambient air in small droplets and aerosols.[10,11] Tight-fitting masks of various weaves and fiber content filter the droplets and aerosols from the air we breathe with various efficiencies.[12] Susceptible uninfected people are protected when the infectious, potentially asymptomatic shedder wears a mask (source control) or when wearing a mask themselves (wearer protection[13]). Every step in this causal chain of reasoning has been researched and documented and has been verified in studies of household transmission of SARS-CoV-2.[14,15]

The exact efficiency of transmission and filtration in each of the stages described can be measured, analyzed, and debated, but it is certainly not zero. From an engineering and materials standpoint, then, the question is not "Do masks work?" but "Do masks work as well as predicted, and if not, why not?" Of course, from immunological, epidemiological, and medical standpoints, we know that there are a host of modifiers that degrade face mask efficacy, including but not limited to the precise relationship between viral shedding and attack rates (i.e., the exact mathematical function connecting number of shed viral particles to number of secondary infections), mask contamination (e.g., wearers touching their masks and then rubbing their eyes), poor fitting around the nose and mouth, compensatory behaviors (mask wearers taking more risks because they think they are better protected than they are), and failure to maintain or use masks properly or at all (which has been a problem in most epidemiological studies of masks). Many of these modifiers contain a component of wearer training and practice, and these suggest that education about proper mask selection, use, and fit are important for improving public protection, as they are directly related to mask efficacy.

Although a detailed look at the Cochrane review demonstrates that the bias, methodological variations, and low adherence to interventions during the studies that were included preclude making firm conclusions about the effects of face masks, modeling the impact of mask wearing on transmission can make the case for masks even if we take the data added to the Cochrane review at face value. In the DANMASK-19 RCT, the authors estimated that no more than 5% of the general population used masks at the time of the study, thus masks were not a significant contribution to source control in the community.[4] The study was not powered to detect a wearer protection efficacy of less than 50%[7] and estimated a confidence interval (CI) ranging from a 46% reduction to a 23% increase in infections for the masked group, so that the effect was not statistically significant. Gurbaxani et al.[3] predicted an approximately 28% to 32% decrease in infections in the masked group, which corroborates the DANMASK-19 measured (but nonsignificant) decrease, although the modeling study assumptions do not closely align with the conditions of the DANMASK-19 study (e.g., the model assumed masks were worn indoors and more widely used in general).

Considering other limitations of the study beyond those discussed, for example, only wearing masks outdoors (where there is much less transmission because of better ventilation), low positive predictive value of testing given low prevalence of SARS-CoV-2 at the time of the study, and potential problems with adherence,[6] the fact that no statistically significant effects were observed for mask wearing was to be expected.

The other new RCT included in the Cochrane review that examined mask wearing to prevent SARS-CoV-2 infection, the Bangladesh RCT,[5] did find a statistically significant, but small, effect for mask wearing. About two orders of magnitude larger than the DANMASK-19 study, the Bangladesh RCT was powered to discern a small effect size and found an 11.5% (95% CI = 6.5%, 17%) reduction in symptomatic illness and 9.5% (95% CI = 1%, 19%) reduction in seropositivity in the masked group compared with the unmasked group.[5] It is notable that some symptomatic individuals did not consent to blood draws, reducing the seropositivity value. The study investigators were able to achieve a 42% adoption of surgical mask (medical procedure mask) wearing in the intervention communities versus 13% in the control communities (with ~180 000 people in each group), which correlated with reductions in seroprevalence.[5]

MODEL CONSISTENCY

The Centers for Disease Control and Prevention (CDC) developed a detailed model that can predict the impact that various levels of masking would have for different types of masks, having measured the filtration efficacy of several different mask types in National Institute for Occupational Safety and Health laboratories.[3,12] The model includes the impact of both symptomatic and asymptomatic transmission; varying degrees of isolation for detected spreaders, including a Bayesian calculation for how well both symptomatic and asymptomatic people are detected; age-structured contact rates; and different levels of masking in each of those compartments.

Plugging the mask adoption rates for the intervention and control communities of the Abaluck et al. study into the model, the model results for reduced infections attributable to mask use are aligned with the Abaluck et al. results.[5] Depending on whether you assume the ancestral virus, or Alpha variant, circulating in Bangladesh at the time of the study (November 2020–April 2021), predictions are for an 8% to 15% drop in infections in the intervention communities (Figure 3 in Gurbaxani et al.[3]; Figure 1 herein). Although some of the parameters used as a default in

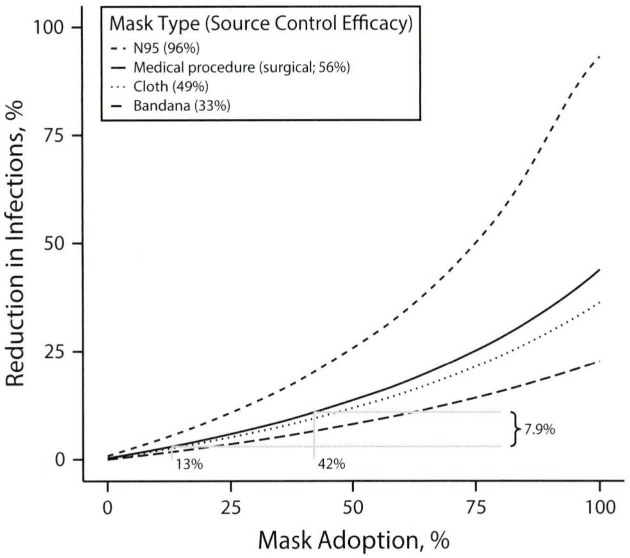

FIGURE 1— Modeled Reduction in SARS-CoV-2 Infections Among the General Population, by Mask Type Relative to No Mask: United States, November 2020–April 2021

Note. The figure shows the percentage reduction in cumulative infections after six months of simulation, relative to no mask use in the population, as mask use varies in the general, susceptible population for different types of face masks (using the model from Gurbaxani et al.[3]). Contact rates between age groups were taken from the POLYMOD study and therefore apply to the US population as of 2017, but other parameters used in the model were taken from a variety of sources[3] and could easily apply to Bangladesh as well as the United States in the 2020–2021 timeframe. Mask source control parameters were fixed according to estimates for the given types, and wearer protection efficacy was assumed to be half of the source control efficacy. Younger susceptible persons were assumed to use masks at 70% of the rate of persons aged 65 years or older. Known infected people aged 65 years or older were masked at a 90% rate, with younger persons at 70%. All parameters were kept the same as similar figures in Gurbaxani et al.,[3] except the baseline basic reproductive number (R_0, the average number of secondary infections resulting from each primary infection) in the absence of mask use was assumed to be 4.0, consistent with the Alpha variant of SARS-CoV-2. Vertical (gray) lines show mask prevalence for medical procedure (surgical) masks in the intervention and control groups of the Abaluck et al.[5] study, and corresponding horizontal lines show the model-predicted reduction in infections over the six-month study period.

the CDC model may or may not match those of the Abaluck et al. study (e.g., the contact rates in the POLYMOD study[16]), the calibration points are in the approximate effect sizes we see in both the DANMASK-19 and the Bangladesh RCT studies. The CDC model also predicts a much higher impact of better-quality masks (e.g., KN95 and KF94 respirators) when used by more than 70% of the population (Gurbaxani et al.[3]; Figure 1), which supports general mask use during times of high transmission to ensure a high population-level impact.

A study by Chikina et al.[17] has suggested that the Bangladesh RCT had an ascertainment bias, which could explain the weak positive result as an artifact of the experiment, given that nearly all of the differences in symptomatic rates between treatment and control groups was attributable to sample size. It is not clear how differences in enrollment and consent at the start of the trial create a significant bias when the outcome is symptomatic seroprevalence at the trial's end, the ratios of which (seropositive to symptomatic) were equal between treatment and control groups. Both Chikina et al.[17] and their publicly available reviewers suggest some possible mechanisms, but these are far from proven. Alternatively, it is quite possible, as Abaluck et al. suggest,[5] that the greater enrollment in the treatment group simply reflected that group's motivation to obtain more masks and the treatment group's surveillance workers' enthusiasm to distribute them. Also, the Chikina et al. article did not address the 23% and 35%, respectively, decreases in symptomatic seroprevalence among the groups aged 50 to 59 years and aged 60 years and older in the intervention group, which cannot be explained by differences in sample size alone and would be expected according to a generally higher symptomatic prevalence for SARS-CoV-2 in those age groups.

Moreover, mask studies inherently suffer from a lack of validation of proper or consistent mask use and of measures of fit and filtration, which would tend to bias the results toward the null hypothesis that masks do not work. Insufficient mask use has been measured even in places where compliance is emphasized and monitored.[18] Either way, neither positive nor negative sources of bias were supported in the Abaluck et al. study. If the Abaluck et al. study proves to be an accurate calibration point for the model, then the widespread use of high-quality, well-fitting masks during times of high transmission shows promise in slowing transmission and reducing the effective reproductive number (R_e).

One of the important criticisms of the Cochrane review is that the role of masks as source control—beyond their role of wearer protection (personal protective equipment)—is an effect that the large RCTs that Cochrane analyzes are not good at estimating.[19] Many types of masks are more effective as source control than they are as wearer protection,[3,12] and, although some have disparaged the distinction,[20] modeling can elucidate the relative impact of source control. In particular, source control is critically important when a respiratory virus is transmitted largely asymptomatically, as seen with SARS-CoV-2.[21]

A modeling study by Glasser et al.,[22] which fit high-quality national serological survey data to a metapopulation model of the spread of the virus, estimated the efficacy of nonpharmaceutical interventions (a combination of masking and social distancing) at 31% in the fall of 2020 (before vaccines were available). Overfitting is not a concern in this estimate, given that the effect of nonpharmaceutical interventions was the only parameter fit to the data in that metapopulation model (see the first table in Glasser et al.[22] for the origin of all the model parameters). This estimate is also in the ballpark of what would be expected given the percentage of cloth and medical procedure mask use in the general population at the time.

MASK EPIDEMIOLOGY BEYOND MODELS

Beyond these modeling validations of the new data added to the Cochrane review of face masks, there are more than a dozen excellent observational epidemiological studies that demonstrate the positive effect of masking, with very sound data and statistical methods, that did not meet the inclusion criteria of the Cochrane framework, which favors large RCTs. Although RCTs are considered ideal, they are not without limitations. Therefore, considering many other data sources along with their strengths and weaknesses is necessary for informed policymaking.[23]

Examples of other studies include that of Donovan et al.,[24] who looked at schools in adjacent school districts in Arkansas—some of which had mask mandates in place, some of which had partial mask mandates, and some of which had none at all—and observed that the strength of the reduction in COVID-19 cases depended on the strength of the mandate, and the results were statistically significant. Other studies of mask mandates showed similar results.[25] Other types of studies, which include controlled laboratory-based experimental studies, epidemiological investigations, and population-level community studies, are detailed in Table A (available as a supplement to the online version of this article at http://www.ajph.org) and merit consideration in assessing the effect of mask use in reducing SARS-CoV-2 transmission.

MORE IS MORE AND BETTER IS BETTER

The science of masking and its impact on SARS-CoV-2 transmission is complicated. Observational studies present valuable data that warrant consideration in informing policy with a full understanding of the utility of mask use in a variety of settings. The Cochrane review did not include a large body of evidence, and that resulted in a biased conclusion. If all types of studies are considered, it is clear that well-fitting, properly used masks do have a measurable and significant effect on reducing transmission when properly worn by the vast majority of the population during times of high community transmission.[3] Although the data in the two new studies included in the Cochrane update on masks are accurate, modeling studies correctly predict the small effect sizes that those studies observed; furthermore, the models predict that the effect size would be much larger with better masks more widely and correctly used. Taken together, these and other studies strongly indicate that masking is an effective intervention to reduce transmission of SARS-CoV-2 (source control) and should be considered to protect those most vulnerable from severe COVID-19 illness (wearer protection) as a general nonpharmaceutical intervention during times of high transmission. AJPH

CORRESPONDENCE

Correspondence should be sent to Brian M. Gurbaxani, Centers for Disease Control and Prevention, 1600 Clifton Rd NE, Bldg 24, 7th Floor, MS H24-7, Atlanta, GA 30333 (e-mail: buw8@cdc.gov). Reprints can be ordered at http://www.ajph.org by clicking the "Reprints" link.

PUBLICATION INFORMATION

Full Citation: Gurbaxani BM, Hill AN, Patel P. Unpacking Cochrane's update on masks and COVID-19. *Am J Public Health*. 2023;113(10):1074–1078.

Acceptance Date: June 25, 2023.

DOI: https://doi.org/10.2105/AJPH.2023.307377

CONTRIBUTORS

B. M. Gurbaxani conceptualized and wrote the initial draft of the article and helped develop the model. A. N. Hill coded the model and script to produce the figure and was the primary modeler. A. N. Hill and P. Patel contributed to article writing. P. Patel added the supplementary material. All authors reviewed and approved the final version.

ACKNOWLEDGMENTS

The authors would like to acknowledge the Centers for Disease Control and Prevention (CDC) COVID-19 incident manager at the time of writing, Brendan Jackson, MD, MPH, and Aron Hall, DVM, MSPH, chief of the Respiratory Viruses Branch, for their support, as well as Rose Wang, MPH, of the Influenza Division for administrative support.

Note. The findings and conclusions in this article are those of the authors and do not necessarily represent the official position of the CDC.

CONFLICTS OF INTEREST

The authors have no conflicts of interest to declare.

REFERENCES

1. Jefferson T, Dooley L, Ferroni E, et al. Physical interventions to interrupt or reduce the spread of respiratory viruses. *Cochrane Database Syst Rev*. 2023;1(1):CD006207. https://doi.org/10.1002/14651858.CD006207.pub6

2. Centers for Disease Control and Prevention. Science brief: community use of masks to control the spread of SARS-CoV-2. February 22, 2022. Available at: https://www.cdc.gov/coronavirus/2019-ncov/science/science-briefs/masking-science-sars-cov2.html. Accessed March 6, 2023.
3. Gurbaxani BM, Hill AN, Paul P, Prasad PV, Slayton RB. Evaluation of different types of face masks to limit the spread of SARS-CoV-2: a modeling study. *Sci Rep.* 2022;12(1):8630. https://doi.org/10.1038/s41598-022-11934-x
4. Bundgaard H, Bundgaard JS, Raaschou-Pedersen DET, et al. Effectiveness of adding a mask recommendation to other public health measures to prevent SARS-CoV-2 infection in Danish mask wearers: a randomized controlled trial. *Ann Intern Med.* 2021;174(3):335–343. https://doi.org/10.7326/M20-6817
5. Abaluck J, Kwong LH, Styczynski A, et al. Impact of community masking on COVID-19: a cluster-randomized trial in Bangladesh. *Science.* 2022;375(6577):eabi9069. https://doi.org/10.1126/science.abi9069
6. Frieden TR, Cash-Goldwasser S. Of masks and methods. *Ann Intern Med.* 2021;174(3):421–422. https://doi.org/10.7326/M20-7499
7. Laine C, Goodman SN, Guallar E. The role of masks in mitigating the SARS-CoV-2 pandemic: another piece of the puzzle. *Ann Intern Med.* 2021;174(3):419–420. https://doi.org/10.7326/M20-7448
8. Cochrane. Statement on physical interventions to interrupt or reduce the spread of respiratory viruses review. March 10, 2023. Available at: https://www.cochrane.org/news/statement-physical-interventions-interrupt-or-reduce-spread-respiratory-viruses-review. Accessed March 14, 2023.
9. Cevik M, Kuppalli K, Kindrachuk J, Peiris M. Virology, transmission, and pathogenesis of SARS-CoV-2. *BMJ.* 2020;371:m3862. https://doi.org/10.1136/bmj.m3862
10. Meselson M. Droplets and aerosols in the transmission of SARS-CoV-2. *N Engl J Med.* 2020;382(21):2063. https://doi.org/10.1056/NEJMc2009324
11. van Doremalen N, Bushmaker T, Morris DH. Aerosol and surface stability of SARS-CoV-2 as compared with SARS-CoV-1. *N Engl J Med.* 2020;382(16):1564–1567. https://doi.org/10.1056/NEJMc2004973
12. Lindsley WG, Blachere FM, Law BF, Beezhold DH, Noti JD. Efficacy of face masks, neck gaiters and face shields for reducing the expulsion of simulated cough-generated aerosols. *Aerosol Sci Technol.* 2021;55(4):449–457. https://doi.org/10.1080/02786826.2020.1862409
13. Ueki H, Furusawa Y, Iwatsuki-Horimoto K, et al. Effectiveness of face masks in preventing airborne transmission of SARS-CoV-2. *mSphere.* 2020;5(5):e00637-20. https://doi.org/10.1128/mSphere.00637-20
14. Centers for Disease Control and Prevention. SARS-CoV-2 B.1.1.529 (Omicron) variant transmission within households—four US jurisdictions, November 2021–February 2022. *MMWR Morb Mortal Wkly Rep.* 2022;71(9):341–346. https://doi.org/10.15585/mmwr.mm7109e1
15. Riley J, Huntley JM, Miller JA, Slaichert ALB, Brown GD. Mask effectiveness for preventing secondary cases of COVID-19, Johnson County, Iowa, USA. *Emerg Infect Dis.* 2022;28(1):69–75. https://doi.org/10.3201/eid2801.211591
16. Prem K, Cook AR, Jit M. Projecting social contact matrices in 152 countries using contact surveys and demographic data. *PLoS Comput Biol.* 2017;13(9):e1005697. https://doi.org/10.1371/journal.pcbi.1005697
17. Chikina M, Pegden W, Recht B. Re-analysis on the statistical sampling biases of a mask promotion trial in Bangladesh: a statistical replication. *Trials.* 2022;23(1):786. https://doi.org/10.1186/s13063-022-06704-z
18. Loyal J, Masub N, Glick SA, Siegel DM. Proper use and compliance of facial masks during the COVID-19 pandemic: an observational study of hospitals in New York City. *Cutis.* 2021;108(6):333–337. https://doi.org/10.12788/cutis.0412
19. MacIntyre CR, Chughtai AA, Fisman D, Greenhalgh T. Yes, masks reduce the risk of spreading COVID—despite a review saying they don't. *The Conversation.* February 6, 2023. Available at: https://theconversation.com/yes-masks-reduce-the-risk-of-spreading-covid-despite-a-review-saying-they-dont-198992. Accessed February 13, 2023.
20. Demasi M. Lead author of new Cochrane review speaks out. February 5, 2023. Available at: https://maryannedemasi.substack.com/p/exclusive-lead-author-of-new-cochrane. Accessed February 21, 2023.
21. Johansson MA, Quandelacy TM, Kada S, et al. SARS-CoV-2 transmission from people without COVID-19 symptoms. *JAMA Netw Open.* 2021;4(1):e2035057. [Erratum in: *JAMA Netw Open.* 2021;4(2):e211383]. https://doi.org/10.1001/jamanetworkopen.2020.35057
22. Glasser JW, Feng Z, Vo M, Jones JN, Clarke KEN. Analysis of serological surveys of antibodies to SARS-CoV-2 in the United States to estimate parameters needed for transmission modeling and to evaluate and improve the accuracy of predictions. *J Theor Biol.* 2023;556:111296. https://doi.org/10.1016/j.jtbi.2022.111296
23. Frieden TR. Evidence for health decision making—beyond randomized, controlled trials. *N Engl J Med.* 2017;377(5):465–475. https://doi.org/10.1056/NEJMra1614394
24. Centers for Disease Control and Prevention. SARS-CoV-2 incidence in K–12 school districts with mask-required versus mask-optional policies—Arkansas, August–October 2021. *MMWR Morb Mortal Wkly Rep.* 2022;71(10):384–389. https://doi.org/10.15585/mmwr.mm7110e1
25. Taylor JD, McCann MH, Richter SJ, Matson D, Robert J. Impact of local mask mandates upon COVID-19 case rates in Oklahoma. *PLoS One.* 2022;17(6):e0269339. https://doi.org/10.1371/journal.pone.0269339

Power Up: A Call for Public Health to Recognize, Analyze, and Shift the Balance in Power Relations to Advance Health and Racial Equity

Jonathan C. Heller, PhD, Paul J. Fleming, PhD, MPH, Ryan J. Petteway, DrPH, MPH, Marjory Givens, PhD, MSPH, and Keshia M. Pollack Porter, PhD, MPH

ABOUT THE AUTHORS

Jonathan C. Heller is with the University of Wisconsin Population Health Institute, Madison, WI, and the National Collaborating Centre for Determinants of Health, Saint Francis Xavier University, Antigonish, Nova Scotia, Canada. Paul J. Fleming is with the University of Michigan School of Public Health, Ann Arbor, MI. Ryan J. Petteway is with the Oregon Health and Science University–Portland State University School of Public Health, Portland, OR. Marjory Givens is with the University of Wisconsin Population Health Institute. Keshia M. Pollack Porter is with the Johns Hopkins Bloomberg School of Public Health, Baltimore, MD.

Strategies such as diversifying the public health workforce; building capacity related to diversity, equity, inclusion, and belonging; and conducting research on oppression are necessary but insufficient to improving health in communities that have been marginalized by systems of oppression. Working toward health and racial equity requires changing the structural drivers of health. Public health interventions must advance widespread and lasting structural change—changes in values and beliefs; culture and norms; governance; laws, policies, regulations, and budgets; and institutional practices.[1]

Structural interventions include, for example, shifting government budgets by increasing taxes on multinational corporations and the wealthy while increasing investment in low-opportunity neighborhoods of color and rural communities. They include changing the US electoral systems to reduce corporate influence, ensuring everyone has a voice that counts equally and can vote freely, and making our elected bodies more democratic and accountable. Structural interventions also include influencing narratives about the virtues of free markets and how the economy works so that the public understands that people govern the economy and can work toward an economy where all can thrive.

Structural interventions require the long-term work of shifting power—both building community power within marginalized communities and contesting the power of those who use it to maintain the status quo. Shifting power means changing who is making public decisions, controlling the political agenda, and influencing dominant narratives. If these are the changes needed to advance equity, does public health currently have the lens, know-how, and audacity to work toward these changes?

Public health needs a power lens: a common, nuanced, and critical understanding of how power works; the potential to mobilize collective power fieldwide; and strategies to shift the balance in power relations to address structural inequity and oppression. We submit that public health must increase its capacity to (1) recognize, (2) analyze, and (3) shift power.

RECOGNIZING POWER

Power remains an underutilized and poorly understood concept in the public health field despite discussion of the topic for decades. Foundational public health frameworks[2,3] and papers[4–6] have described power as a fundamental cause of health inequities and balancing power as an important strategy in advancing health equity, yet those ideas have not been widely integrated into research and practice. Public health research has shown that power imbalance explains inequities across multiple determinants of health, though this insight has been muddied by overlapping terminology, such as "control" and "autonomy."[7] Some in public health have developed and applied frameworks for analyzing power.[8,9] Despite this, a power lens is rarely applied.

Useful frameworks for conceptualizing power can inform how the field

AJPH October 2023, Vol 113, No. 10

recognizes power. Feminist scholars and activists have introduced concepts such as power to, power with, and power within, considering power to be a capacity or a resource that can be redistributed.[10] Social theorist Steven Lukes described power as having three "faces."[11] As described elsewhere, these are (1) "Exercising influence in the political or public arena and amongst formal decision-making bodies to achieve a particular outcome"; (2) "Organizing the decision-making environment, including who can access decision-making and what issues are being considered by decision-making bodies"; and (3) "Shaping information, beliefs and worldviews about social issues."[12(p35)]

Black feminist sociologist Patricia Hill Collins articulated four domains of power: (1) structural: the social structures, such as laws, religion, and the economy, that organize power relations and maintain oppression; (2) disciplinary: control and organization of behavior through surveillance and routinization to manage oppression; (3) hegemonic: the shaping of beliefs through the development and normalization of ideology and culture to legitimize oppression; and (4) interpersonal: the personal relationships and interactions that are part of our daily life that uphold oppression.[13]

Each component of these conceptualizations is readily discernible in public health's external research and interventions and in its internal workings, with implications for public health training, research, practice, funding, publishing, and accreditation. As a first step, public health professionals can study these frameworks, critically reflect on how power is relevant to our work, and embed a recognition of power into our training and practice.

ANALYZING POWER

Theoretical descriptions of power are most useful when they can guide research, policy, and practice, such as through the development and answering of questions that prompt analyses of power dynamics. For example, questions that can guide public health analysis based on the "three faces of power" include the following:

1. Who holds decision-making power? How do we influence them? What public health assets (e.g., evidence, framing) will influence them?
2. Who is influencing the decision-making agenda? What organizations need to be built or brought into relationship to move an equity agenda?
3. What dominant worldviews and narratives influence decisions and make harmful viewpoints seem like common sense? What transformative narratives can public health and partners in marginalized communities assert to shift what is considered common sense?

Similarly, questions can be developed from Hill's four domains of power. Examples relevant to public health training include the following:

1. Structural: What are the present and historical relationships between school or program of public health (SPPH) property ownership and land acquisition practices and community housing, and what have been and are the health impacts for residents? How are the SPPH's labor practices assessed and addressed? Are SPPH staff, faculty, and research and teaching assistants paid fairly?
2. Disciplinary: How is power operating to shape public health epistemologies and training requirements? How are various domains and types of knowledge valued within admissions criteria? Which forms of knowledge and ways of knowing are emphasized, prioritized, and centered?
3. Hegemonic: How is power operating in the determination of public health training competencies? Are accreditation entities and program directors sufficiently trained in matters of positionality, power, epistemology, and the social production of knowledge? Do curricula presume public health is an "objective" and "neutral" arbiter of facts, evidence, and health "truths"?
4. Interpersonal: How is power operating to support or inhibit inclusion and belonging within SPPHs? Are there policies in place to disrupt practices of silencing, erasure, and microaggressions in public health classrooms?

Using frameworks of power to develop and answer questions about the power dynamics at play on issues related to health equity is a second step for public health.

SHIFTING THE BALANCE IN POWER RELATIONS

While some may conceive of power as dominance—power over—Dr Martin Luther King Jr defined power more affirmatively as "the ability to achieve purpose."[14(p199)] To advance equity, power must be shifted from those who use power to perpetuate inequity. This requires contesting their power as well as building power with and within marginalized communities.

Answers to the types of questions outlined previously must inform the strategic actions and interventions public health deploys to advance equity. While some in public health are already intentionally working to shift power—for example, using the "three faces" framework[12]—for many, this will mean working differently and starting new activities.

Public health will need to shift the balance in power relations through its community interventions. For example, public health departments can provide services while also building power among those they serve, bringing together marginalized individuals and communities to build relationships, develop a shared understanding of the root causes of the issues they face, and work together to identify and advance solutions that address those root causes. Through Health in All Policies and similar initiatives, public health can engage across sectors to build a shared understanding of equity and support work across sectors to shift power. Every aspect of our community work can be evaluated and shifted through a power lens: What public health assets and actions can be mobilized to grow power within marginalized communities to influence decisions, build the infrastructure necessary to set an equity-focused agenda, and change the narrative?

Shifting power will require new relationships and collaborations—for example, with community organizing groups that have long focused on shifting power to marginalized communities. It will require that public health researchers ask how research contributes to power-building and shift to more inclusive methods such as participatory research.[15] Public health will need to reconsider what is viewed as legitimate data and research, how knowledge is assessed and validated, and how to challenge dominant narratives that block progress toward structural change.[16]

To enable this externally facing work, public health practitioners will need to examine our own power and positionality, understanding the power we have and how it can be harnessed to advance equity. Public health organizations will need to transform institutional practices, critically examining processes for research, funding, publishing, administration, and training.[16] Public health training will need to reorient around advocacy, social action, and political engagement, and abandon teaching that we are "objective" and "neutral" arbiters of science.

Increasingly, public health practitioners recognize that to advance health and racial equity we must change the structures that cause and maintain inequity, addressing structural racism and other structures of oppression. Yet methods and interventions for making those changes are absent from public health's current toolbox. Using a power lens can reveal a way forward. The field of public health must learn to recognize and analyze power, harness our collective capacity, and change our strategies to correct power imbalances. AJPH

CORRESPONDENCE

Correspondence should be sent to Jonathan C. Heller, UW Population Health Institute, 610 Walnut St, 575 WARF, Madison, WI 53726 (e-mail: jheller7@wisc.edu). Reprints can be ordered at https://ajph.org by clicking the "Reprints" link.

PUBLICATION INFORMATION

Full Citation: Heller JC, Fleming PJ, Petteway RJ, Givens M, Pollack Porter KM. Power up: a call for public health to recognize, analyze, and shift the balance in power relations to advance health and racial equity. *Am J Public Health.* 2023;113(10): 1079–1082.

Acceptance Date: June 28, 2023.

DOI: https://doi.org/10.2105/AJPH.2023.307380

CONTRIBUTORS

J. C. Heller conceptualized this article, wrote the first draft, and oversaw the editing and review process. P. J. Fleming, R. J. Petteway, M. Givens, and K. M. Pollack Porter contributed conceptual elements, writing and editing, and review.

ACKNOWLEDGMENTS

This work was supported in part by grant funding from the W. K. Kellogg Foundation and the Robert Wood Johnson Foundation.

Note. The views expressed here do not necessarily reflect the views of the funders.

CONFLICTS OF INTEREST

The authors report no conflicts of interest.

REFERENCES

1. Solar O, Irwin A. A conceptual framework for action on the social determinants of health. World Health Organization Commission on the Social Determinants of Health. 2010. Available at: https://www.who.int/publications-detail-redirect/9789241500852. Accessed October 13, 2022.
2. World Health Organization. The Ottawa Charter for Health Promotion. 1986. Available at: https://www.who.int/publications/i/item/ottawa-charter-for-health-promotion. Accessed November 16, 2021.
3. Closing the gap in a generation: health equity through action on the social determinants of health. World Health Organization Commission on the Social Determinants of Health. 2008. Available at: https://www.who.int/publications-detail-redirect/WHO-IER-CSDH-08.1. Accessed November 16, 2021.
4. Link BG, Phelan J. Social conditions as fundamental causes of disease. *J Health Soc Behav.* 1995; (spec no.):80–94. https://doi.org/10.2307/2626958
5. Waitzkin H. A Marxist view of medical care. *Ann Intern Med.* 1978;89(2):264–278. https://doi.org/10.7326/0003-4819-89-2-264
6. Beckfield J, Krieger N. Epi + demos + cracy: linking political systems and priorities to the magnitude of health inequities—evidence, gaps, and a research agenda. *Epidemiol Rev.* 2009;31(1): 152–177. https://doi.org/10.1093/epirev/mxp002
7. Iton A, Ross RK, Tamber PS. Building community power to dismantle policy-based structural inequity in population health. *Health Aff (Millwood).* 2022;41(12):1763–1771. https://doi.org/10.1377/hlthaff.2022.00540
8. Popay J, Whitehead M, Ponsford R, Egan M, Mead R. Power, control, communities and health inequalities I: theories, concepts and analytical frameworks. *Health Promot Int.* 2021;36(5): 1253–1263. https://doi.org/10.1093/heapro/daaa133

9. Friel S, Townsend B, Fisher M, Harris P, Freeman T, Baum F. Power and the people's health. *Soc Sci Med.* 2021;282:114173. https://doi.org/10.1016/j.socscimed.2021.114173
10. Allen A. Feminist perspectives on power. In: Zalta EN, ed. *The Stanford Encyclopedia of Philosophy.* 2022. Available at: https://plato.stanford.edu/archives/fall2022/entries/feminist-power. Accessed November 30, 2022.
11. Lukes S. *Power: A Radical View.* 3rd ed. New York, NY: Bloomsbury Publishing; 2021.
12. Heller JC, Little OM, Faust V, et al. Theory in action: public health and community power building for health equity. *J Public Health Manag Pract.* 2023;29(1):33–38. https://doi.org/10.1097/PHH.0000000000001681
13. Collins PH. *Feminist Thought: Knowledge, Consciousness, and the Politics of Empowerment.* London, UK: Routledge Classics; 1991.
14. King ML Jr. *The Essential Martin Luther King, Jr.: "I Have a Dream" and Other Great Writings.* Boston, MA: Beacon Press; 2013.
15. Fleming PJ, Stone LC, Creary MS, et al. Antiracism and community-based participatory research: synergies, challenges, and opportunities. *Am J Public Health.* 2023;113(1):70–78. https://doi.org/10.2105/AJPH.2022.307114
16. Petteway RJ. On epidemiology as racial-capitalist (re)colonization and epistemic violence. *Crit Public Health.* 2022;33(1):5–12. https://doi.org/10.1080/09581596.2022.2107486

Time to End Racial Disparities in Buprenorphine Access

Henry Rosen, MS, and Chinazo O. Cunningham, MD, MS

ABOUT THE AUTHORS

Henry Rosen is the Chief of Staff at the New York State Office of Addiction Services and Supports, New York, NY. Chinazo O. Cunningham is the Commissioner of the New York State Office of Addiction Services and Supports and is a clinical professor of medicine at the Albert Einstein College of Medicine, New York, NY.

On December 29, 2022, US President Joe Biden signed the Consolidated Appropriations Act of 2023, which eliminated the Drug Abuse Treatment Act of 2000 (DATA 2000) waiver requirement, commonly called the "X-waiver" requirement. This change to US drug policy means qualified providers can now prescribe buprenorphine, one of three medications that effectively treat opioid use disorder (OUD), without first obtaining an X-waiver.[1]

The X-waiver was a barrier to expanding access to buprenorphine treatment of OUD. Ending the X-waiver requirement could reshape medical treatment of OUD and help stem the course of the US drug overdose epidemic.[2] Importantly, it also presents an opportunity for government officials and health and public health practitioners to redress the harms of policies that disproportionately affect low-income communities and Black, Indigenous, and other People of Color (BIPOC).

RACIAL DISPARITIES IN DRUG OVERDOSE IN THE UNITED STATES

Nationally, drug overdose deaths have increased markedly since the late 1990s, with some of the most pronounced increases occurring over the last decade. The epidemic has comprised three waves: starting in the 1990s, the first wave was an epidemic of prescription opioid overdose; starting in 2010, the second wave was marked by an increase in heroin-involved overdose deaths; and beginning in 2013, the third wave has been characterized by a drastic increase in overdose deaths driven by synthetic opioids, primarily fentanyl.[3] During each wave, the burden of overdose deaths has not been distributed evenly and has varied across race/ethnicity, gender, geography, and neighborhood-level wealth or income.[3,4]

Although overdose deaths have increased among all racial and ethnic groups over the last few years, overdose death rates were highest or have grown most in many BIPOC communities.[4–7] In 2021, age-adjusted overdose death rates were highest among non-Hispanic American Indian or Alaska Native persons (56.6 deaths per 100 000 people), followed by non-Hispanic Black persons (44.2 deaths per 100 000 people). From 2020 to 2021, the relative rate increase in overdose deaths among Hispanic persons (20%) was nearly double that of White persons (11%).[5]

Recent data also show that drug overdose rates increase as county-level income inequalities increase. From 2019 to 2020, non-Hispanic Black persons and Hispanic persons experienced the greatest burden of drug overdose deaths in communities with high income inequalities.[8]

Lastly, a history of substance use treatment was lowest among non-Hispanic Black, Hispanic, and non-Hispanic American Indian or Alaska Native decedents, groups that have experienced some of the greatest increases in drug overdose death rates.[8]

Consistent with causes of other health inequities, the disproportionate burden of overdose deaths in BIPOC communities is the result of decades-long, racist social policies and failed drug policies that structurally disadvantage and harm BIPOC communities.[4,9,10]

DISPARATE ACCESS TO MEDICATIONS TO TREAT OPIOID USE DISORDER

Of the three medications approved for OUD treatment, methadone and buprenorphine are most commonly prescribed and both are effective at reducing opioid use, improving treatment retention, and reducing risk of overdose death.[11] Despite these benefits, both medications are carefully regulated to prevent diversion and, particularly in the case of methadone, misuse. The regulatory structures, however, have contributed to wide disparities in accessibility along geographic, socioeconomic, and racial and ethnic lines.[7,12]

Methadone for OUD treatment can only be prescribed and administered in specialized addiction treatment settings known as opioid treatment programs. Typically, people who are taking methadone must go to an opioid

AJPH October 2023, Vol 113, No. 10

treatment program nearly daily to be administered a single dose under observation but can sometimes receive multiday doses at the discretion of a provider. In contrast to methadone, buprenorphine for OUD treatment can be administered and prescribed by providers (previously, only by X-waivered providers) in any setting, with medication dispensed by community pharmacies.[12]

Although the X-waiver requirement was designed to expand access to buprenorphine for OUD outside opioid treatment program settings, it created several restrictions.[13] To become waivered, a provider needed to complete eight to 24 hours of additional training as well as satisfy other administrative requirements. These requirements were a considerable hurdle, and partially explain the low numbers of waivered prescribers.[2,7,13] DATA 2000 also imposed limits on the number of patients that waivered providers could treat, and these limits could only be increased if providers submitted an application at least one year after receiving their waiver. These limits further constrained access to buprenorphine for OUD.[2,7,13]

In addition to the X-waiver requirement, several other factors discouraged providers from obtaining an X-waiver, prescribing buprenorphine once waivered, or treating the maximum allowable number of patients. These factors include concerns related to financial costs and compensation, a lack of institutional support, concerns about taking on OUD patients without additional training and support, and stigmatizing beliefs about people who use drugs or have OUD.[2,7,14]

Issues of stigma and racism have also been shown to deter engagement into treatment among BIPOC patients. Black patients delay seeking addiction treatment as a result of both previously experiencing racism and anticipating racial discrimination in health care settings, including the addiction treatment system,[15] where addiction physicians and psychiatrists are predominantly White.[16] These findings are consistent with the corpus of literature that shows how racism and lack of racial and cultural concordance drive poorer access, treatment, and health outcomes among BIPOC patients compared with their White counterparts.[15]

Unsurprising in this context, among providers with X-waivers, most serve White, middle- and upper-income communities, and only about half accept public insurance. Even among commercial insurance beneficiaries, Black and Hispanic patients are less likely to receive buprenorphine than White patients.[7,17] And, although the Affordable Care Act helped expand access to OUD treatment with both buprenorphine and methadone, buprenorphine remained comparatively inaccessible in BIPOC communities.[18]

In part driven by the regulatory environment, buprenorphine has been far more accessible to whiter and wealthier communities, yet BIPOC communities and communities experiencing poverty have less access to buprenorphine and much greater access to methadone. The benefits of receiving buprenorphine treatment have not been evenly distributed and have failed to keep pace with the growing number of people with OUD.[7]

LOOKING FORWARD

Elimination of the X-waiver is a cause for rejoicing among clinicians, addiction experts, advocates, people who use drugs and their loved ones, public health professionals, and policymakers alike. It is an important step toward expanding access to OUD treatment, an urgent need at a time when drug overdose deaths have reached historically high numbers. It also represents a long-overdue step toward advancing health equity and addressing the structural racism deeply embedded in US drug policies as well as in the US health care system.

As others have noted,[19] and as history has shown, reducing regulatory barriers alone is unlikely to close the gaps between the need for and availability of OUD treatment, particularly the treatment gaps that exist along racial and ethnic divisions. It is unlikely that the removal of the X-waiver alone will generate large numbers of new prescribers nor grow existing prescriber caseloads. However, research has shed light on the need for other regulatory changes as well as the need for more provider education, training, and support. With one major obstacle out of the way, it is therefore incumbent upon health care providers, public health practitioners, and policymakers to implement new strategies to make buprenorphine readily available and attractive to those who want or need it; it is also critical that these strategies prioritize racial equity and serve to undo the effects of decades-long, de facto medical redlining policies. AJPH

CORRESPONDENCE

Correspondence should be sent to Henry Rosen, MS, New York State Office of Addiction Services and Supports, 501 7th Ave, 8th Fl, New York, NY 10018 (e-mail: Henry.Rosen@oasas.ny.gov). Reprints can be ordered at http://www.ajph.org by clicking the "Reprints" link.

PUBLICATION INFORMATION

Full Citation: Rosen H, Cunningham CO. Time to end racial disparities in buprenorphine access. *Am J Public Health*. 2023;113(10):1083–1085.

Acceptance Date: July 7, 2023.

DOI: https://doi.org/10.2105/AJPH.2023.307388

CONTRIBUTORS

H. Rosen conceptualized the manuscript and led the writing. C. O. Cunningham conceptualized the manuscript and contributed to the writing.

CONFLICTS OF INTEREST

The authors have no conflicts of interest to disclose.

REFERENCES

1. Substance Abuse and Mental Health Services Administration. Medications for substance use disorders. Updated February 21, 2023. Available at: https://www.samhsa.gov/medications-substance-use-disorders/removal-data-waiver-requirement. Accessed March 13, 2023.
2. Woodruff AE, Tomanovich M, Beletsky L, Salisbury-Afshar E, Wakeman S, Ostrovsky A. Dismantling buprenorphine policy can provide more comprehensive addiction treatment. *NAM Perspect.* 2019: 10.31478/201909a. https://doi.org/10.31478/201909a
3. Lippold K, Ali B. Racial/ethnic differences in opioid-involved overdose deaths across metropolitan and non-metropolitan areas in the United States, 1999–2017. *Drug Alcohol Depend.* 2020; 212:108059. https://doi.org/10.1016/j.drugalcdep.2020.108059
4. Friedman J, Hansen H. Far from a "white problem": responding to the overdose crisis as a racial justice issue. *Am J Public Health.* 2022;112(suppl 1): S30–S32. https://doi.org/10.2105/AJPH.2021.306698
5. Spencer MR, Miniño AM, Warner M. *Drug Overdose Deaths in the United States, 2001–2021.* Hyattsville, MD: National Center for Health Statistics; 2022. NCHS Data Brief no. 457. https://dx.doi.org/10.15620/cdc:122556
6. Furr-Holden D, Milam AJ, Wang L, Sadler R. African Americans now outpace whites in opioid-involved overdose deaths: a comparison of temporal trends from 1999 to 2018. *Addiction.* 2021;116(3):677–683. https://doi.org/10.1111/add.15233
7. Guerrero EG, Amaro H, Khachikian T, Zahir M, Marsh JC. A bifurcated opioid treatment system and widening insidious disparities. *Addict Behav.* 2022;130:107296. https://doi.org/10.1016/j.addbeh.2022.107296
8. Kariisa M, Davis NL, Kumar S, et al. Vital signs: drug overdose deaths, by selected sociodemographic and social determinants of health characteristics—25 states and the District of Columbia, 2019–2020. *MMWR Morb Mortal Wkly Rep.* 2022;71(29):940–947. https://doi.org/10.15585/mmwr.mm7129e2
9. Jurecka CA, Barocas JA. Using evidence to inform legislation aimed at curbing fentanyl deaths. *JAMA Health Forum.* 2023;4(1):e225202. https://doi.org/10.1001/jamahealthforum.2022.5202
10. Kunins HV. Structural racism and the opioid overdose epidemic: the need for antiracist public health practice. *J Public Health Manag Pract.* 2020;26(3):201–205. https://doi.org/10.1097/PHH.0000000000001168
11. Volkow ND, Frieden TR, Hyde PS, et al. Medication-assisted therapies: tackling the opioid-overdose epidemic. *N Engl J Med.* 2014;370(22):2063–2066. https://doi.org/10.1056/NEJMp1402780
12. US Government Accountability Office. Opioid addiction: laws, regulations, and other factors can affect medication-assisted treatment access. September 2016. GAO-16-833. Available at: https://www.gao.gov/products/gao-16-833. Accessed February 13, 2023.
13. Lanham HJ, Papac J, Olmos DI, et al. Survey of barriers and facilitators to prescribing buprenorphine and clinician perceptions on the Drug Addiction Treatment Act of 2000 Waiver. *JAMA Netw Open.* 2022;5(5):e2212419. https://doi.org/10.1001/jamanetworkopen.2022.12419
14. Louie DL, Assefa MT, McGovern MP. Attitudes of primary care physicians toward prescribing buprenorphine: a narrative review. *BMC Fam Pract.* 2019;20(1):157. https://doi.org/10.1186/s12875-019-1047-z
15. Hall OT, Bhadra-Heintz NM, Teater J, et al. Group-based medical mistrust and care expectations among Black patients seeking addiction treatment. *Drug Alcohol Depend Rep.* 2022;2:100026. https://doi.org/10.1016/j.dadr.2022.100026
16. Garcia ME, Coffman J, Jordan A, Martin M. Lack of racial and ethnic diversity among addiction physicians. *J Gen Intern Med.* 2022;37(12):3214–3216. https://doi.org/10.1007/s11606-022-07405-8
17. Lagisetty PA, Ross R, Bohnert A, Clay M, Maust DT. Buprenorphine treatment divide by race/ethnicity and payment. *JAMA Psychiatry.* 2019;76(9):979–981. https://doi.org/10.1001/jamapsychiatry.2019.0876
18. Hansen HB, Siegel CE, Case BG, et al. Variation in use of buprenorphine and methadone treatment by racial, ethnic, and income characteristics of residential social areas in New York City. *J Behav Health Serv Res.* 2013;40(3):367–377. https://doi.org/10.1007/s11414-013-9341-3
19. Larson C. It's not "magic": ending the X-waiver alone unlikely to fix MAT's access problem. Behavioral Health Business. March 3, 2023. Available at: https://bhbusiness.com/2023/03/03/its-not-magic-ending-the-X-waiver-alone-unlikely-to-fix-mats-access-problem. Published and Accessed March 3, 2023.

FORWARD: Building a Model to Hold Schools of Public Health Accountable for Antiracism Work

Samantha Garbers, PhD, MPA, Michael A. Joseph, PhD, Bethany Jankunis, JD, MSW, Maria O'Brien, MBA, MPH, and Linda P. Fried, MD, MPH

Schools of public health have increasingly adopted programs, praxis, and competencies for antiracist work. Fighting Oppression, Racism and White Supremacy through Action, Research and Discourse (FORWARD) was founded to accelerate antiracist work at the Columbia University Mailman School of Public Health in New York City. Seven action corps reporting to an accountability cabinet were established with 183 participants. FORWARD achieved progress across five core pillars. We describe how an iterative, dynamic structure and explicit framework for accountability can guide future antiracism work. (*Am J Public Health*. 2023;113(10):1086–1088. https://doi.org/10.2105/AJPH.2023.307356)

AJPH October 2023, Vol 113, No. 10

Working to eradicate health inequities is central to the mission of public health. Schools of public health have focused on issues of diversity, inclusion, and belonging, but there is a need for initiatives that more directly address structural racism rooted in White supremacy that systematically disadvantages Black people, Indigenous people, and other people of color (BIPOC).[1,2] In schools of public health, a lack of representation of people from diverse backgrounds and lived experiences reflects systematic exclusion that hinders the advancement of the field.[3,4]

INTERVENTION AND IMPLEMENTATION

The Fighting Oppression, Racism and White Supremacy through Action, Research and Discourse (FORWARD) initiative (https://bit.ly/3PxfuMl) was established at Columbia University's Mailman School of Public Health to accelerate the school's transformation into an antiracist, multicultural, and fully inclusive institution in all aspects of its culture and operations; to create shared vision, goals, and leadership in dismantling the toxic structures that continue to sustain racism and health inequities; and to create a positive, supportive, and inclusive environment for all. FORWARD, with a mandate to coordinate and complement existing structures and serve as a community engagement mechanism with an explicit antiracist lens, was founded in 2020 as a school-wide initiative under the auspices of the dean's office.

Research indicates that antiracism initiatives are particularly effective when they are evidence based, are long term focused, and include ongoing rigorous evaluation.[5] FORWARD was intentionally designed to have a dynamic, proactive (vs reactive) organizational structure to support sustained engagement across constituencies in and beyond the institution. FORWARD's structure reflects features of continuous quality improvement[6] (Figure A [available as a supplement to the online version of this article at http://www.ajph.org] incorporates evidence of effective features of antiracism initiatives).[5,7]

PLACE, TIME, AND PERSONS

FORWARD was established by the dean and leaders of offices in Columbia University Mailman School of Public Health, a predominantly White institution in New York City with 1400 students (48% racial or ethnic minority from 52 countries), 363 faculty members, and 549 administrators and officers.

FORWARD was formed to propose and coordinate antiracist work, engage members of the school community across functions and disciplines, and facilitate collaboration and communication across structures involved directly and indirectly with activities related to FORWARD's vision, including human resources; offices of diversity, culture, and inclusion; career services; enrollment management; and educational initiatives.

The central hub of FORWARD is an 18-member accountability cabinet reporting to the dean, which plays a key role in the initiative's iterative structure, establishing action corps each year (Figure A). In years 1 and 2, seven action corps served as the primary mechanism through which activities and accountability planning, consistent with their charges (Table A, available as a supplement to the online version of this article at http://www.ajph.org), were carried out. Action corps are managed by two coleaders, generally faculty and middle- to senior-level administrators. Volunteer participants are allocated across action corps with an eye to representation by constituency (i.e., faculty, staff, students, alumni); diversity, equity, and inclusion experience; and administrative structure affiliation. FORWARD's work is advisory to the dean.

Action corps had 183 participants in years 1 and 2. In year 2, following active recruitment, 39 alumni participated (Table A). Action corps met monthly or more often, with workgroups engaged between meetings. At year end, each action corps presented to the accountability cabinet 3 to 5 recommended next steps (called "Fast FORWARDS"). Recommendations included establishing funded student fellowships to support FORWARD goals and conducting a full curriculum review. The accountability cabinet elevated priorities to the dean for agreement, implementation, and funding and delineated charges for subsequent action corps.

Because FORWARD's programmatic work (Table A, "Charge" column) is carried out by volunteers, institutional investment in staffing at the administrative and leadership levels was made. Each action corps partnered with a project manager, who synthesized internal data and current work in the school and university, identified promising approaches and best practices to recommend, shared successful strategies and lessons learned across action corps, and developed communications strategies.

PURPOSE

Eliminating the structural roots of racism requires long-term effective interventions. FORWARD's first two years focused on short-term goals to catalyze subsequent cycles of continuous improvement, theorizing that small-scale initial successes will help the initiative to demonstrate progress and gain traction. FORWARD established core pillars of the initiative, representing the short-term goals for each of the initiative's structural levels (Table B, available as a supplement to the online version of this article at http://www.ajph.org). These pillars reflect the institution's stakeholders (i.e., students, faculty, staff, alumni, leadership, members of the community [i.e., the New York City neighborhoods of Washington Heights, Inwood, and Harlem]) and serve as a framework for accountability and evaluation.

EVALUATION AND ADVERSE EFFECTS

The Goals and Measuring Progress Action Corps operationalized each pillar statement to elucidate the short- and longer-term goals and identified indicators to evaluate progress across each pillar. Table B summarizes the pillars' operationalization and progress made the first two years.

Programmatic initiatives have been consistently approved and funded. Direct FORWARD investments by the dean (years 1–2) included administrative (i.e., project management, communications, and other support; one full-time equivalent) and leadership (one quarter full-time equivalent) salary support, direct research support, annual stipends for five students engaging in community work and six FORWARD fellows, antiracism training and speaker fees, and mentoring program expansion. This did not include substantial indirect investments and joint investments with offices.

SUSTAINABILITY

Operating in a large institution and relying on overburdened volunteer members present sustainability challenges. Ongoing, cyclical monitoring and evaluation build in opportunities to reflect on progress, recognize contributions, and identify next steps.[7] A transparent accountability mechanism is a key responsibility for institutions that seek to improve health, including through antiracist work. Adapting a continuous quality improvement framework further supports a dynamic long-term focus (Figure A).[5]

Building interdisciplinary teams with faculty, staff, students, and alumni to conduct this work is key. Using a multidisciplinary and multiperspective structure with alumni and staff as coequals with faculty and students builds community, preserves continuity over time, offers opportunities to build trust and identify mutual goals, and breaks down silos for joint work on charges (Table A). Formal institutional investment in program management support uses the programmatic work of the action corps, supports sustained engagement of volunteer participants, and minimizes

AJPH October 2023, Vol 113, No. 10

gaps in progress caused by competing priorities of action corps participants.

PUBLIC HEALTH SIGNIFICANCE

Training public health students in racial justice and health equity is an essential part of public health education,[8] but it is not sufficient.[9] The antiracist work of schools of public health is also accountable to faculty, staff, alumni, and the communities in which the school resides and with whom the school works.[10] Predominantly White institutions must confront, examine, and change the systems that have historically excluded or disadvantaged BIPOC and other minoritized or marginalized individuals and work at all levels to dismantle these systems. This work requires a paradigm shift, but to date, there has been little guidance on how initiatives should be structured. We have described the mechanisms through which a school of public health can carry out antiracist work with a sustained commitment through an iterative, dynamic structure with committed leadership and school-wide participation and an explicit statement of, and framework for, accountability.

This review of FORWARD's inception and structure can guide replication at other schools of public health. The process of an antiracist initiative is as important as the outcomes: nurturing an environment where participants of all backgrounds feel comfortable sharing their perspectives is critically important.[2] FORWARD's structure is designed to acknowledge and mitigate issues of power and positionality[11,12] by fostering formal and informal connections as diverse teams work together in and across action corps, catalyzing full participation across the institution's constituencies.[5] Future work must explore how this initiative has changed the school's culture, activities, and outcomes. AJPH

ABOUT THE AUTHORS

Samantha Garbers is with the Heilbrunn Department of Population & Family Health, Columbia University Mailman School of Public Health, New York, NY. Michael A. Joseph, Bethany Jankunis, Maria O'Brien, and Linda P. Fried are with the Dean's Office, Columbia University Mailman School of Public Health.

CORRESPONDENCE

Correspondence should be sent to Samantha Garbers, PhD, Associate Professor, Heilbrunn Department of Population & Family Health, Columbia University Mailman School of Public Health, 60 Haven Ave, Room B3-311, New York, NY 10032 (e-mail: svg2108@cumc.columbia.edu). Reprints can be ordered at http://www.ajph.org by clicking the "Reprints" link.

PUBLICATION INFORMATION

Full Citation: Garbers S, Joseph MA, Jankunis B, O'Brien M, Fried LP. FORWARD: building a model to hold schools of public health accountable for antiracism work. *Am J Public Health*. 2023; 113(10):1086–1088.

Acceptance Date: May 23, 2023.

DOI: https://doi.org/10.2105/AJPH.2023.307356

CONTRIBUTORS

S. Garbers led the drafting, information synthesis, and writing. M. A. Joseph and L. P. Fried conceptualized the scope of the article. B. Jankunis and M. O'Brien contributed significant information on the development of the initiative and contributed to the conceptualization of the article's scope. All authors participated in writing and editing.

ACKNOWLEDGMENTS

The authors acknowledge the essential contributions of the members of the accountability cabinet and action corps; program managers, including G. Capone, Christina Ferrari, Leisa Herrera, Westley Holiday, and Lauren Sagnella; and Dorcas Adedoja, Daniel Alohan, Charles Branas, Raygine DiAquoi, Clare Norton, and Maggie Wiggin.

CONFLICTS OF INTEREST

The authors have no conflicts of interests to declare.

HUMAN PARTICIPANT PROTECTION

No protocol approval was necessary because this study was not designated as human participants research. All data used were obtained in aggregate.

REFERENCES

1. Merino Y. What do schools of public health have to say about diversity and inclusion? *Pedagogy Health Promot*. 2019;5(4):233–240. https://doi.org/10.1177/2373379918811820
2. Alang S, Hardeman R, Karbeah J, et al. White supremacy and the core functions of public health. *Am J Public Health*. 2021;111(5):815–819. https://doi.org/10.2105/AJPH.2020.306137
3. Abraído-Lanza AF, Echeverria SE, Flórez KR, Mendoza-Grey S. Latina women in academia: challenges and opportunities. *Front Public Health*. 2022;10:966. https://doi.org/10.3389/fpubh.2022.876161
4. Goodman MS, Plepys CM, Bather JR, Kelliher RM, Healton CG. Racial/ethnic diversity in academic public health: 20-year update. *Public Health Rep*. 2020;135(1):74–81. https://doi.org/10.1177/0033354919887747
5. Ben J, Kelly D, Paradies Y. Contemporary anti-racism: a review of effective practice. In: Solomos J, ed., *Routledge International Handbook of Contemporary Racisms*. London, England: Routledge; 2020:205–215.
6. Rubenstein L, Khodyakov D, Hempel S, et al. How can we recognize continuous quality improvement? *Int J Qual Health Care*. 2014;26(1):6–15. https://doi.org/10.1093/intqhc/mzt085
7. Hassen N, Lofters A, Michael S, Mall A, Pinto AD, Rackal J. Implementing anti-racism interventions in healthcare settings: a scoping review. *Int J Environ Res Public Health*. 2021;18(6):2993. https://doi.org/10.3390/ijerph18062993
8. Chandler CE, Williams CR, Turner MW, Shanahan ME. Training public health students in racial justice and health equity: a systematic review. *Public Health Rep*. 2022;137(2):375–385. https://doi.org/10.1177/00333549211015665
9. Tsui EK, Huynh M. Combating anti-Asian American/Pacific Islander racism through local health departments and schools of public health. *Am J Public Health*. 2021;111(8):1470–1472. https://doi.org/10.2105/AJPH.2021.306391
10. Levin MB, Bowie JV, Ragsdale SK, Gawad AL, Cooper LA, Sharfstein JM. Enhancing community engagement by schools and programs of public health in the United States. *Annu Rev Public Health*. 2021;42:405–421. https://doi.org/10.1146/annurev-publhealth-090419-102324
11. Fried LP, Begg MD, Bayer R, Galea S. MPH education for the 21st century: motivation, rationale, and key principles for the new Columbia public health curriculum. *Am J Public Health*. 2014;104(1):23–30. https://doi.org/10.2105/AJPH.2013.301399
12. Aqil AR, Malik M, Jacques KA, et al. Engaging in anti-oppressive public health teaching: challenges and recommendations. *Pedagogy Health Promot*. 2021;7(4):344–353. https://doi.org/10.1177/23733799211045407

Integrated COVID-19 Interventions in a Native American Community: Arizona, December 25, 2021–January 31, 2022

Elizabeth A. Van Dyne, MD, MPH, Christopher Jentoft, MD, Thomas Boone, MD, and Ryan M. Close, MD, MPH

COVID-19 has disproportionately affected Indigenous communities. The Whiteriver Service Unit (WRSU) took an integrated public health–health care system delivery approach in collaboration with the White Mountain Apache Tribe to decrease the case fatality rate (CFR). The WRSU performed daily data analyses identifying risk factors, expeditiously treating and proactively vaccinating people during at-home visits. The WRSU's CFR was 0.3% lower than Arizona's ($P = .04$). Among communities disproportionally affected, an integrated approach using data to drive real-time decision-making among a culturally competent workforce can contribute to decreased CFR. (*Am J Public Health*. 2023;113(10):1089–1092. https://doi.org/10.2105/AJPH.2023.307364)

AJPH October 2023, Vol 113, No. 10

During the December 2021–April 2022 COVID-19 surge, the Department of Preventative Medicine (DPM) of the Indian Health Service's Whiteriver Service Unit (WRSU) built upon and strengthened existing local processes to coordinate care across various public health and clinical teams, importantly involving community members, to mitigate the impact of disease. Real-time, data-driven, and efficiently communicated decisions allowed a nimble response embedded in the community that streamlined case identification, individual patient risk assessment, and early linkage to care and vaccination.

INTERVENTION AND IMPLEMENTATION

After the first community COVID-19 case was detected on April 1, 2020, the WRSU's DPM coordinated the response to COVID-19, developing the high-risk team, contact tracing, case investigation, COVID-19 vaccination program, and high-risk home visit teams. The WRSU used a single, integrated electronic health record system for the DPM, ambulatory and inpatient care, the emergency department (ED), and community outreach. The DPM comprises physicians, nurses, medical assistants, pharmacists, physical therapists, health technicians, dental hygienists, and community health representatives performing public health system roles.

During the COVID-19 omicron (B.1.1.529 and descendant lineages) surge that began in December 2021, the DPM daily obtained laboratory COVID-19 test results, performed analyses to create reports of all positive results, and identified persons at increased risk for progression to severe disease, based on age, underlying conditions, and vaccination status. These persons were monitored at home visits (history, ambulatory and resting pulse oximetry, physical exam) and remotely (self-monitored pulse oximetry). Those who met specific, locally developed criteria were referred to the WRSU's ED for further evaluation.

The high-risk team reviewed the electronic health record of all patients who tested positive for COVID-19 to determine eligibility for early treatment with either monoclonal antibody or other antiviral medication (sotrovimab, combined casirivimab and imdevimab, and remdesivir) based on the Food and Drug Administration's Emergency Use Authorization and locally defined criteria. The WRSU developed a specific scoring system (the COVID-19 Treatment Allocation Score), adapting external allocation systems (Monoclonal

Allocation Screening Score and National Institutes of Health COVID-19 Treatment Guidelines Panel) based on local data and outcomes. These criteria were updated in real time through an Incident Command System, necessitated by the rapid influx of patients during the surge of cases. The COVID-19 Treatment Allocation Score was used to identify patients to contact for treatment, not to exclude patients from treatment; individual clinicians had independent authority to order treatments for patients based on individual, case-based, clinical discretion.

The WRSU engaged in aggressive, proactive COVID-19 vaccine efforts. Field team members, many of whom were from the community and spoke the local language, provided home vaccinations for persons at increased risk. Hospital-wide patient encounters were reviewed to identify opportunities to provide vaccination to prevent future surges.

PLACE, TIME, AND PERSONS

The WRSU serves approximately 18 000 members of the White Mountain Apache Tribe (WMAT) and other tribes on the reservation and surrounding areas across approximately 2600 square miles in remote and mountainous east-central Arizona. During January 2022, 97% of test samples for SARS-CoV-2 (the virus that causes COVID-19) sequenced in Arizona were BA.1 omicron variant.[1] The WRSU and WMAT faced the highest case rates of the entire pandemic among a high-risk population remote from intensive care unit–level care (180 miles from nearest tertiary care centers). On December 20, 2021, near the start of the state omicron surge, the COVID-19 Pandemic Vulnerability Index of Navajo County, Arizona (where WMAT is located) was higher than those of 97% of US counties, predictive of higher incidence and mortality risk.[2] Arizona experienced the highest weekly case count of the entire pandemic (2.4 times the previous highest weekly case count for the state) and less than 5% intensive care unit bed availability.[3,4]

PURPOSE

Native American communities endured great morbidity and mortality from the COVID-19 pandemic; in Arizona, 13% of COVID-19 cases and 18% of deaths were among Native Americans, who make up only 5.3% of the state's population.[3,5,6] To decrease the case fatality rate (CFR) and offer culturally competent care, the WRSU implemented a proactive COVID-19 risk management strategy, integrating public health, preventive medicine, and health care delivery.

EVALUATION AND ADVERSE EFFECTS

During the BA.1 omicron surge (December 25, 2021–January 31, 2022), the COVID-19 CFR in the WRSU was significantly lower than that in the rest of Arizona. Despite a 69% higher COVID-19 incidence (incidence rate ratio [IRR] = 1.69; $P \le .001$), the CFR in the WRSU (0.14%) was one third that in Arizona overall (0.44%).[7,8] These outcomes are notable; Indigenous communities have been disproportionately affected by COVID-19 with mortality rates consistently higher than the US average.[9]

A total of 2168 persons in the WRSU catchment area (12 044 per 100 000) received a positive SARS-CoV-2 test result (Table 1). Among these, 41 patients (1.9%) were hospitalized (228 per 100 000), and three patients (0.14%) died. Compared with Arizona, where the COVID-19 incidence was 7136 per 100 000, the WRSU incidence was significantly higher (IRR = 1.69) and correlates with the higher county COVID-19 Pandemic Vulnerability Index. The overall Arizona CFR (0.44%) was more than three times that of the WRSU (CFR difference = −0.3; $P = .04$). COVID-19–related mortality among WRSU patients (17 per 100 000) was 47% lower than that in Arizona overall (32 per 100 000), although the difference was not statistically significant (IRR = 0.53; $P = .26$).

Among 1616 persons aged 18 years or older with a positive SARS-CoV-2 test result, 528 (33%) received treatment, including 319 (20%), 186 (12%), and 23 (1%) who received sotrovimab, combined casirivimab and imdevimab, and a three-day outpatient course of remdesivir, respectively (Table 2). Of three WRSU deaths among patients with laboratory-confirmed COVID-19, none met Emergency Use Authorization criteria for outpatient treatment because of oxygen requirements or hospitalization at time of diagnosis. Among patients who received any outpatient treatment, no deaths occurred.

In a review of patient encounters to assess opportunities to deliver COVID-19 vaccine, it was found that 75% of patients seen in the ED in January 2022 were not up to date. ED-based vaccinations were initiated by pharmacists to avoid relying on ED staff to administer vaccines.

SUSTAINABILITY

The WRSU's DPM, which coordinated and conducted the WRSU community COVID-19 response, has full-time staff and will continue to use the same

TABLE 1— COVID-19 Cases and Outcomes: Whiteriver Service Unit (WRSU) and Arizona, December 25, 2021–January 31, 2022

	No. (Rate per 100 000)		
Characteristic	WRSU[a]	State of Arizona[b]	IRR (95% CI)
Cases of confirmed COVID-19	2 168 (12 044)	519 431 (7 139)	1.69 (1.62, 1.76)
COVID-19–related hospitalizations	41 (228)	16 245 (223)	1.02 (0.73, 1.39)
COVID-19–related deaths	3 (17)	2 294 (32)	0.53 (0.11, 1.55)
Case fatality rate, % (95% CI)[c]	0.14 (−0.02, 0.30)	0.44 (0.42, 0.46)	. . .

Note. CI = confidence interval; IRR = incidence rate ratio.

[a]Rates per 100 000 were calculated for cases, hospitalizations, and deaths using the electronic health record (EHR) for WRSU population-level data. The Indian Health Service EHR, in conjunction with iCare, a population management software tool, and Resource and Patient Management System, were used for WRSU data collection for health care delivery and public health analyses and decision-making.
[b]Trends in number of COVID-19 cases and deaths in the United States by state/territory, as reported to the Centers for Disease Control and Prevention (CDC), were accessed by data download from https://covid.cdc.gov/covid-data-tracker/#trends_dailycases, https://covid.cdc.gov/covid-data-tracker/#cases_totaldeaths, and https://covid.cdc.gov/covid-data-tracker/#new-hospital-admissions (accessed October 11, 2022). The CDC calculates the number of new cases or deaths each day either by using the information provided by states and territorial jurisdictions or by calculating the difference in cumulative counts reported by the state from the day before. Rates per 100 000 are calculated as total cases or deaths per 100 000 people using the US Census Bureau Population Estimates Program.
[c]Case fatality rate difference between WRSU and Arizona was −0.30 percentage points (95% CI = −0.46, −0.14; $P = .04$).

strategy to respond to other diseases. The WRSU coordinates with tribal government agencies (e.g., the Emergency Operations Committee, the Public Health Department, community health representatives, and the WMAT Emergency Medical Services) to enhance sustainability.

TABLE 2— COVID-19 Treatment Outcomes Among Persons Aged ≥ 18 Years With a Positive SARS-CoV-2 Test Result: Whiteriver Service Unit, Arizona, December 25, 2021–January 31, 2022

Treatment Outcome	No. (%)
Total with positive SARS-CoV-2 test result	1616 (100)
Received outpatient treatment[a]	528 (33)
Sotrovimab	319 (20)
Casirivimab/imdevimab	186 (12)
Remdesivir	23 (1)
Death	0
Did not receive outpatient treatment	1088 (67)
Met EUA criteria for outpatient treatment[b]	1032 (64)
Did not meet EUA criteria[c]	56 (3)
Death	3 (0.2)

Note. EUA = Food and Drug Administration's Emergency Use Authorization.

[a]Treatment included sotrovimab, casirivimab/imdevimab, or remdesivir.
[b]Patients categorized as high risk and who met EUA criteria for outpatient treatment.
[c]Patients who required oxygen therapy because of COVID-19, were hospitalized because of COVID-19, or otherwise did not meet EUA criteria for outpatient treatment.

PUBLIC HEALTH SIGNIFICANCE

The WRSU's COVID-19 response demonstrates how an integrated, proactive approach using data to drive dynamic, real-time decision-making among a dedicated workforce that understands the local community context, can contribute to a decreased CFR.[10] Clear and real-time communication was essential to the response, particularly in meeting time-frame goals for treatments.

Home outreach can require substantial investments of time and human resources; however, in this remote population with limited resources, including transportation, as well as limited or unavailable Internet and video capabilities, there were few other alternatives to reaching persons at highest risk for severe disease. In addition, seeing patients in their own environment and performing a physical examination provide more information than can be obtained through a telephone call, inform clinical decision-making, and enhance patient care. Early identification of patients at high risk, streamlining expedient treatment, and linking to ongoing care through home visits all contributed to improvements in outcomes. Preemptive planning of vaccination efforts while still in surge mitigation phase has the potential to reduce future morbidity and mortality.

A proactive risk management and health strategy, preventive measures, collaborative and integrative interventions involving health care and public health institutions from the community to hospital level, and an integrated data-driven response led to a COVID-19 CFR that was significantly lower than that of the rest of Arizona. Among communities disproportionally affected by COVID-19, an integrated approach using data to drive dynamic, real-time decision-making among a culturally competent workforce can contribute to decreased COVID-19 case fatality. AJPH

ABOUT THE AUTHORS

Elizabeth A. Van Dyne is with the US Public Health Service Commissioned Corps and Food Safety and Inspection Service, US Department of Agriculture, Tucson, AZ. Christopher Jentoft, Thomas Boone, and Ryan M. Close are with Whiteriver Indian Hospital, Indian Health Service, Whiteriver, AZ.

CORRESPONDENCE

Correspondence should be sent to Elizabeth A. Van Dyne, 2000 East Allen Rd, Tucson, AZ 85719 (e-mail: Elizabeth.VanDyne@usda.gov). Reprints can be ordered at http://www.ajph.org by clicking the "Reprints" link.

PUBLICATION INFORMATION

Full Citation: Van Dyne EA, Jentoft C, Boone T, Close RM. Integrated COVID-19 interventions in a Native American community: Arizona, December 25, 2021–January 31, 2022. *Am J Public Health*. 2023;113(10):1089–1092.

Acceptance Date: June 10, 2023.

DOI: https://doi.org/10.2105/AJPH.2023.307364

CONTRIBUTORS

E. A. Van Dyne and R. M. Close performed conceptualization, data analysis, and interpretation of data, and drafted and edited the article. C. Jentoft performed conceptualization and interpretation of data, and drafted and edited the article. T. Boone performed data analysis, and drafted and edited the article.

ACKNOWLEDGMENTS

We thank WMAT Tribal Chairwoman Gwendena Lee-Gatewood, the WMAT Tribal Council, the WMAT Emergency Operations Center, J. T. Nasio and WMAT Community Health Representative Program, the Whiteriver Service Unit Department of Preventative Medicine, the US Public Health Service Commissioned Corps officers deployed to the Whiteriver Service Unit for COVID-19, and all Whiteriver Service Unit leadership and employees.

CONFLICTS OF INTEREST

The authors report no potential conflicts of interest.

HUMAN PARTICIPANT PROTECTION

Data and article were reviewed and approved by the WMAT Tribal Health Advisory Board and the WMAT Tribal Council.

REFERENCES

1. Translational Genomics Research Institute. Arizona COVID-19 Sequencing Dashboard. Available at: https://pathogen.tgen.org/covidseq-tracker. Accessed April 8, 2022.
2. National Institutes of Health, National Institute of Environmental Health Sciences. COVID-19 Pandemic Vulnerability Index (PVI): PVI Model (12/20/2021), model 11. 2. Available at: https://covid19pvi.niehs.nih.gov. Accessed April 8, 2022.
3. Arizona Dept of Health Services. COVID-19 cases by week. Available at: https://www.azdhs.gov/covid19/data/index.php#confirmed-by-week. Accessed April 8, 2022.
4. Arizona Dept of Health Services. Hospital bed usage & availability. Available at: https://www.azdhs.gov/covid19/data/index.php#hospital-bed-usage. Accessed April 8, 2022.
5. Tai DBG, Shah A, Doubeni CA, Sia IG, Wieland ML. The disproportionate impact of COVID-19 on racial and ethnic minorities in the United States. *Clin Infect Dis*. 2021;72(4):703–706. https://doi.org/10.1093/cid/ciaa815
6. US Census Bureau. Census Bureau QuickFacts. Arizona. 2018. Available at: https://www.census.gov/quickfacts/fact/table/AZ/PST045218. Accessed April 28, 2020.
7. Close RM, Jones TS, Jentoft C, McAuley JB. Outcome comparison of high-risk Native American patients who did or did not receive monoclonal antibody treatment for COVID-19. *JAMA Netw Open*. 2021;4:e2125866. https://doi.org/10.1001/jamanetworkopen.2021.25866
8. Stone MJ, Close RM, Jentoft CK, et al. High-risk outreach for COVID-19 mortality reduction in an indigenous community. *Am J Public Health*. 2021;111:1939–1141. https://doi.org/10.2105/AJPH.2021.306472
9. Arrazola J, Masiello MM, Joshi S, et al. COVID-19 mortality among American Indian and Alaska Native persons—14 states, January–June 2020. *MMWR Morb Mortal Wkly Rep*. 2020;69(49):1853–1856. https://doi.org/10.15585/mmwr.mm6949a3
10. Emanuel EJ, Osterholm M, Gounder CR. Strategy for the "new normal" of life with COVID—reply. *JAMA*. 2022;327(18):1824. https://doi.org/10.1001/jama.2022.4305

On Building Common Ground: An *AJPH* Special Section

Michael Fine, MD, William J. Kassler, MD, MPH, and Tanya Telfair LeBlanc, PhD, MS

ABOUT THE AUTHORS

Michael Fine is with the City of Central Falls, RI. He was director of the Rhode Island Department of Health, 2011–2015. William Kassler was the state health officer and medical director of the New Hampshire Department of Health and Human Services, 1998–2005. Tanya Telfair LeBlanc is an AJPH *associate editor.*

See also Building Common Ground, pp. 1093–1115.

Protecting the health and safety of all Americans depends on at least three capacities: the ability to determine how health and safety is best protected scientifically; the ability to communicate the logic, risks, and benefits of proposed interventions so the population trusts the interventions suggested; and the ability to convene communities so that they see the need for these interventions as part of the common good. Building common ground has become more challenging as the nation struggles to see itself as one people. The roles of public health and of public health leadership in building that common ground have always been implicit, but the increasing polarization of the nation requires a more conscious effort from public health and public health leadership if we are to be effective in protecting the health and safety of all Americans.

In public health, "finding common ground" is commonly applied to subject matter related to racial/ethnic diversity, equity, and inclusion. The world and the United States are diverse places whether we acknowledge and embrace diversity, equity, and inclusion or not. Too often in the United States, we are sorted or sort ourselves by income, education, race, faith, gender preference, and geography, and too many of us exist in bubbles: a social environment where we know and interact only with people with whom we share some common identifier. Consequently, we often exist without encountering ideas and beliefs different from our own, and too often we have no context in which to learn about or appreciate the ideas of others.[1]

In the special section "Building Common Ground," *AJPH* offers a new paradigm—suggestions for expanding the notion of diversity to include diversity of thought and perspectives built from lived experiences, frames of references, and differing worldviews—with the goal of forming public health strategies for public good in a landscape of varied political, cultural, and ideological perspectives. We hope to open dialogues on these challenging issues, identify points of articulation among persons with differing worldviews, and locate best practices that help us come to agreement on how to best promote population health.

Honest and transparent communication is critical in this endeavor, as are mutual respect, understanding and fairness, and tolerance of differing ideas. We acknowledge the specific challenges of cultivating common ground in the United States, with our tiered governmental structures (i.e., the local, state, and federal levels), which sometimes serve as barriers to accomplishments, as well as our well-documented difficulty in transcending the usual variety of competing interest groups and seeing ourselves as Americans, unified for the common good. We conceptualize this special section as an open door to continuing conversations in incremental steps to identify methodologies, strategies, and practices that will facilitate building common ground, brick by brick, and learning along the journey.

When a group of our colleagues who are Association of State and Territorial Health Officials alumni, former state health officers who served in both Republican and Democratic administrations, proposed a special section on building common ground, we were uncertain what building common ground would entail. But the process of putting out a call for articles, reading the submissions, and determining which submissions best fit our developing criteria helped us understand both the need for common ground and the skills, knowledge, and wisdom required in creating that common ground.

Our call for proposals asked for articles on building an understanding among groups with differing viewpoints, values, ideologies, or perspectives to better address programs, policies, and interventions in public health and population health. We determined that building common ground occurs when different people or groups find areas of policy or programmatic agreement, even when they do not agree about ideology,

AJPH October 2023, Vol 113, No. 10

policy, or politics. We understood that, although building common ground has always been challenging in public health policy, the current political and ideological division in the United States (and indeed the world) has reached levels that threaten progress in many domains. But we also understood that public health and population health improvement presents many opportunities to build common ground to produce better population health outcomes.

The Comments, Notes From the Field, and Editorials in this special section represent a first-pass attempt to address the opportunities presented to public health as a convener and facilitator of the process to find common ground in this one aspect of US policy, culture, and society, as we focus on the consensus necessary to protect the health and safety of all Americans.

Telfair LeBlanc (p. 1096) reflects on contemporary trends in the quantity and quality of available information and on the distortion of public confidence in information created by spin and social media. She recommends that schools of public health design specific courses to create awareness of the information conundrum to help future public health professionals discern fact from fiction and clearly differentiate between conclusions based on opinions and those based on empirical evidence.

Kassler and Bowman (p. 1102) question the now sometimes fraught language of public health surveillance and expose how our legitimate desire for privacy makes that language a wedge that threatens our common ground. They propose ways to change the programs and systems we develop to emphasize the same high priority for privacy and civil liberties that our policymakers and their constituents demand so that our language will resonate among all.

Bernier (p. 1099) reports on the Crosscurrents Dialogue Model, which has been used to explore how Americans with different political perspectives can have productive conversations about controversial value-laden topics. He suggests that the divide among Americans can be narrowed by the Crosscurrents Dialogue Model enough to reach agreement on public health interventions.

Similarly, Blacksher et al. (p. 1110) describe public deliberation, a process that convenes people of varied backgrounds to learn and talk together about a social problem in search of solutions. They describe the core principles and practices of deliberation, provide examples of its use in the health sector, discuss deliberation design adaptations attuned to a divided and diverse United States, and describe where and how it could be used to address decision making in US population health.

Magnan and Kindig (p. 1106) share 12 principles that may be helpful in fostering agreements about public health issues and ideas among people who may not agree about other things.

Finally, Alberti et al. (p. 1114), writing from the Association of American Medical Colleges Center for Health Justice, report on a nationally representative poll of 1510 members of Generation Z: those aged 18 to 24 years. The poll identified unexpected areas of agreement among these younger self-identified Democrats, Independents, and Republicans, and the results give us hope for a future focused on health equity that builds those areas of agreement.

We hope that this special section will further the development of this public health skill set and that we see many other articles, reports, and editorials as we develop science based on the approach to building common ground but also knowledge and wisdom based on the science. We hope future articles (and, perhaps, future special sections) will tell the stories of successful and unsuccessful attempts to build common ground, highlighting best practices and using rigorous evaluation methodology. Such articles will name the convener, the major parties to the process, and their positions and differences; the processes used to reach common ground; the processes used to maintain negotiating equipoise; the intervention chosen; the methodology by which that intervention was successful; and the results achieved. The articles will also discuss lessons learned and thoughts about scalability.

The common ground we find and build in public health is necessary for public health to succeed in protecting the health and safety of all Americans. That common ground is part of a bigger picture—a perception of our membership in one nation, indivisible after all, which is likely a necessary condition for democracy and for a better, safer, and stronger future. AJPH

CORRESPONDENCE

Correspondence should be sent to Michael Fine, MD, 348 Gleaner Chapel Rd, Scituate, RI (e-mail: michaelfinemd@gmail.com). Reprints can be ordered at http://www.ajph.org by clicking the "Reprints" link.

PUBLICATION INFORMATION

Full Citation: Fine M, Kassler WJ, LeBlanc TT. On building common ground: an *AJPH* special section. *Am J Public Health*. 2023;113(10):1093–1095.

Acceptance Date: July 19, 2023.

DOI: https://doi.org/10.2105/AJPH.2023.307399

CONTRIBUTORS

M. Fine drafted the editorial. W. J. Kassler and T. T. LeBlanc made editorial suggestions. T. T. LeBlanc added to the original draft. All authors helped conceptualize the editorial and the special section.

ACKNOWLEDGMENTS

The authors gratefully acknowledge our Association of State and Territorial Health Officials alumni colleagues, particularly those who helped draft the call for submissions; all who submitted contributions in response to the call for submissions; the reviewers; and the *AJPH* editorial staff.

CONFLICTS OF INTEREST

The authors have no conflicts of interest to declare.

REFERENCE

1. Bishop W. *The Big Sort. Why the Clustering of Like-Minded America Is Tearing Us Apart.* New York, NY: Houghton Mifflin; 2008.

Quality and (Un)Certainty of Information: A Critical Concern for Building Common Ground

Tanya Telfair LeBlanc, PhD, MS

ABOUT THE AUTHOR

Tanya Telfair LeBlanc is an AJPH associate editor.

See also Building Common Ground, pp. 1093–1115.

Forging common ground among the disparate entities involved in protecting the public's health is confounded by contemporary trends in the quantity and quality of available information and public confidence in information.

We are only 23 years into the 21st century, but life for ordinary people, especially those in the United States, has changed significantly during the period. The "information age," which employs computers, the Internet, smartphones, tablets, and other electronic devices, eases access to countless content products and applications—in seconds rather than hours. The rapidity of information dissemination has many advantages. Results of medical tests can be interpreted rapidly to aid in speedier diagnosis and treatment of illnesses. College students and professionals are able to conduct literature searches online in minutes, rather than days. Many people born in the 2000s and later have likely never heard of a library card catalog or read a hard copy newspaper.

TROUBLING MEDIA TRENDS

However, mass media trends that began in the 1990s have evolved to alter how people receive, understand, interpret, and internalize all kinds of information. Those trends include (1) use of spin in broadcast and print media, (2) segmentation of media markets and creation of media silos, and (3) the rise of social media platforms.

Technically, "spin" is defined as "the selective assembly of facts and the shaping of nuance to support a particular view of a story" (https://bit.ly/44C7Zs6). Although the origin of the concept dates to decades earlier, the concept of spin became popular in public parlance in the 1990s during a number of political scandals and debates. Use of the term was essential in the context of cable television and 24-hour news cycles, which had become normative in the American experience.

The 24-hour news cycle, which repeated the same stories over and over again, required a fresh take on reporting each time it aired. Obsession with following news stories, in the same way some people follow soap operas, and absorbing incremental updates as the saga goes on and on, are common. People have become obsessed with following media content, anticipating breaking news. Crafting the interpretation of facts to fit a political persuasion or ideological perspective has become the norm in news reporting.

Many young people today may have never experienced consistent factual reporting of current events by all television and online news outlets in the way Walter Cronkite anchored for the *CBS Evening News* and NBC's anchor team did on the *Huntley–Brinkley Report*. In the current news landscape, if one were to use the line Cronkite ended his broadcasts with—"and that's the way it is"—one would have to add a qualifier such as "that depends."

DIMINISHED RELEVANCE OF FACTS

Building on spin, news outlets have become increasingly partisan and ideological, with the emergence of segmented media markets and silos catering to specific perspectives and interpretations of events. News consumers can select outlets interpreting current events through lenses of personal ideological or political biases, which have become more entrenched in dogma and extreme over time. The segmentation of media outlets has influenced the phenomenon of "truth decay." Truth decay is described as the diminished role that verifiable facts, credible data, and accurate analysis play in everyday informal, political, and civil discourse, and especially in news reporting. The RAND Corporation highlights four related trends undergirding truth decay:

> (1) increasing disagreement about facts, (2) the blurring of the line between opinion and fact, (3) the increasing volume and influence of opinion over fact, and (4) declining trust in formerly respected sources of fact.[1(p2)]

The distortion of facts is further complicated by the growth of Internet use, which opened the opportunity for any person, anywhere to obtain a Web address, develop a credible-appearing Web site, and post articles that appear to present news or analyses.

The understanding of truth then for many persons who consume news through television, radio, and online media hubs is not always based on empirically verifiable facts. Rather, what is accepted as truth is generally partisan or ideological perspective spin carefully crafted to trigger emotional responses with the goal of stimulating the consumer to some action. Discerning between fact and fiction has become more complex, as conveyors of media content use misinformation, disinformation, nuance, and hyperbole to influence purchasing merchandise, voting for a political candidate, contributing to a political campaign, perceiving imagined threats, and, in extreme cases, committing violent acts.

CONCENTRATED PERSPECTIVES

Into this troubling cauldron of burgeoning information misuse and distortion comes the social media phenomenon. Although the earliest forms of social media, which experienced limited popularity, were actually developed in the 1990s, the trendsetting MySpace and later Facebook, Twitter, and YouTube emerged in the 2000s, unleashing a tidal wave of global popularity. These interactive applications allowed any user to create and share content around the world in seconds. Facebook, which became one of the most popular social media platforms, started as a university student–only platform at Harvard, spread to other colleges internationally, and spread later to the general public.

At first use of these technologies, friends from high school or college could reconnect, and family members living across the country or the globe could share news of weddings and births. Grandparents could receive pictures of grandchildren, immediately enjoying hallmarks of their developing years, which would otherwise be lost to geographical distancing. However, with the opportunities to monetize access to millions of social media users and marketing products based on the use of registering "likes" (approval of content), these companies realized enormous profits from advertising revenue. Algorithms, which channel content based on approval of specific topics, were eventually applied to further concentrate types of content among specific users. This trend exacerbated the siloing of information on social media, giving users an increasing volume of political and cultural perspectives like their own.

At least one published study demonstrated Facebooks' ability to stir powerful emotions, either positive or negative, among users, termed "emotional contagion" by the authors.[2] Information shared on social media has evolved into a potent tool for extreme galvanization of users with hardened "us versus them" perspectives and demonization of persons with differing ideation. Importantly, social media spreads misinformation and disinformation for profit and can be used to manipulate the opinions of and evoke powerful emotions in individuals who do not seek information elsewhere or from credible sources.[3]

Add to these phenomena the fact that, according to a 2021 Pew Research Center survey, fewer Americans are obtaining information from books (https://bit.ly/471iWVW).

The trilogy of media trends, (1) use of spin, (2) the segmentation of media markets and media silos, and (3) the rise of social media platforms has confounded dissemination of credible information in science and in public health—two essential institutions that directly affect population well-being. We saw observable evidence of fact distortion and confusion during the COVID-19 pandemic, which likely contributed to unnecessary morbidity and mortality. In the interest of finding common ground to solve complex public health problems, including disparities in maternal and infant mortality, widespread incidence of chronic diseases, and the next pandemic, those of us who work in science and public health must seek ways to counter the media trends that contribute to and support a hardening of political and cultural perspectives that serve to entrench individuals into imagined communities built on a shared distortion of facts. To prepare for coping with these realities, schools of public health should consider developing specific courses designed to create awareness of the information conundrum, help future public health professionals discern fact from fiction, and clearly differentiate between conclusions based on opinions from those based on empirical evidence. AJPH

CORRESPONDENCE

Correspondence should be sent to Tanya Telfair LeBlanc, 800 I Street, NW, Washington, DC 20001 (e-mail: ttantelfair@gmail.com). Reprints can be ordered at http://www.ajph.org by clicking the "Reprints" link.

PUBLICATION INFORMATION

Full Citation: LeBlanc TT. Quality and (un)certainty of information: a critical concern for building common ground. *Am J Public Health*. 2023;113(10): 1096–1098.

Acceptance Date: July 18, 2023.

DOI: https://doi.org/10.2105/AJPH.2023.307397

ACKNOWLEDGMENTS

I would like to thank Alfredo Morabia, *AJPH* editor-in-chief, for offering the opportunity to co-guest edit the Common Ground special section with William Kassler and Michael Fine.

CONFLICTS OF INTEREST

The author has no conflicts of interest to declare.

REFERENCES

1. Williams HJ, McCulloch C. *Truth Decay and National Security Intersections, Insights, and Questions for Future Research.* Santa Monica, CA: RAND Corporation; 2023.
2. Kramer AD, Guillory JE, Hancock JT. Experimental evidence of massive-scale emotional contagion through social networks. *Proc Natl Acad Sci U S A.* 2014;111(24):8788–8790. https://doi.org/10.1073/pnas.1320040111. [Expression of concern in: Verma IM. Editorial expression of concern: experimental evidence of massive-scale emotional contagion through social networks. *Proc Natl Acad Sci U S A.* 2014;111(29):10779. https://doi.org/10.1073/pnas.1412583111.]
3. Oates S. The easy weaponization of social media: why profit has trumped security for US companies. *Digi War.* 2020;1(1–3):117–122. https://doi.org/10.1057/s42984-020-00012-z

The Crosscurrents Dialogue Model: 2019–2023

Roger H. Bernier, PhD, MPH

See also Building Common Ground, pp. 1093–1115.

The failure to consult with the public in policymaking can result in less sound and supportable policies. The Crosscurrents Dialogue Model (CDM) was developed to explore if Americans with different political perspectives could have useful policy conversations. To date, the CDM participants have addressed 10 separate topics such as health care and immigration and reached agreements each time. CDM provides evidence that the divide between politically diverse Americans can be bridged adequately to agree on specific recommendations for action. (*Am J Public Health*. 2023;113(10):1099–1101. https://doi.org/10.2105/AJPH.2023.307359)

The politicization of public health interventions in the United States during the COVID-19 pandemic helped make clear what has always been true but not often acknowledged publicly. Namely, public health is politics.[1] The frequently heard advice for policymakers to just "follow the science" has never been an adequate guide for action because the facts do not just speak for themselves. Behind most public health and other public policy choices are competing social values,[2] and decision-makers in public health have often relied largely on their own values or those of expert committees in making public policy decisions. Since our core values as Americans reside in the body politic, the failure to meaningfully consult with the public on values tradeoffs in arriving at evidence-informed decisions can result in less sound, less values-aligned, and less supportable public policies.

Critiques of the US pandemic response are now calling for more community engagement in developing public health policies.[3,4] However, the deep political polarization that now characterizes American society raises questions about how to effectively engage with populations that harbor diverse and strongly held views, not just on vaccines, masks, and lockdowns but on myriad other topics as well.

INTERVENTION AND IMPLEMENTATION

The Crosscurrents Dialogue Model (CDM) is a small-group problem-solving methodology used to explore whether everyday Americans with different political values could have frank conversations about timely, controversial topics and reach agreement on recommendations for addressing the problems. Both health and nonhealth topics were selected for discussion. CDM overlaps with the use of a charette method, which also involves problem-solving, but most often the charette topics center on planning and design choices rather than public policy options.

PLACE, TIME, AND PERSONS

The CDM was implemented in Beaufort and Aiken counties in South Carolina beginning in 2019. Meetings were carried out in person or via videoconferencing for approximately two hours every two weeks and have continued uninterrupted for three years, including during the pandemic. The group started with two liberal and two conservative persons at a breakfast meeting and has grown to attract an estimated 50 different individuals of different ages, races, and genders with an average of between 10 and 15 members at any given point in time. The membership has consistently included people representing diverse political views. Prerequisites for joining the group are curiosity, the capacity to be open-minded, and an interest in learning from others. During the meetings, the ground rules agreed upon are to avoid dominating the discussion, to be respectful, and, when disagreeing, to do so inoffensively. A member of the group serves as moderator and organizer.

To date, members have met on separate topics of gun control, impeachment, health care reform, election reform, police reform, the

AJPH October 2023, Vol 113, No. 10

existence of shared public values, immigration, threats to democracy, civil discourse, and teaching American history. For each topic, members gathered relevant facts from reliable sources, discussed competing values and different points of view, found shared interests or common ground, identified practical solutions, and agreed on recommendations.

PURPOSE

The motivation for the intervention is to provide "proof of concept" that individuals with very diverse political views can have productive dialogues. The goal is achieved by publishing the agreements in local newspapers so that the conversations can serve as an example to other citizens and public officials of what can be accomplished through dialogue.

EVALUATION AND ADVERSE EFFECTS

To date, the CDM has made it possible for diverse Americans to reach 12 separate agreements on 10 different topics. Each agreement has been on a limited set of actions that could be taken to better address the public problem. Each of these agreements has been submitted and published by local newspapers covering four towns in two counties of South Carolina. The publication of the group's agreements has led to the recruitment of new members who have helped to sustain the desired average number of participants. Also, the publicity about the CDM has led to other groups organizing to use the model in new areas. For example, the CDM has been piloted by the Osher Lifelong Learning Institute at the University of South Carolina Beaufort,[5] and a modified version has been carried out by interested dialogue practitioners in Northeastern Ohio.[6] There have been no adverse or unintended consequences associated with CDM.

SUSTAINABILITY

The CDM has been in continuous use for three years and has tackled numerous different topics with a continuous turnover of regular members leaving and new members joining. The new members have been attracted after reading one or more of the published statements and learning about the group. The project demonstrates that there is a public appetite for safe spaces and proven effective methods for exchanging views and learning from other citizens who think differently.

PUBLIC HEALTH SIGNIFICANCE

Many reports describing lessons learned from the recent pandemic call for greater community engagement to develop more effective and supportable public health interventions.[3,4] Most calls are for the involvement of like-minded stakeholders who already support the public health mission. Few calls for community engagement highlight the need for involvement of citizens with diverse political persuasions. We found no reports that provide convincing evidence that it will be possible for public health officials to bridge the chasm that now separates Americans. Admittedly, the CDM has not produced any major changes in the fundamental political perspectives of participants. However, those unchanged worldviews have not been an obstacle to reaching agreement on specific recommendations to help solve the problem discussed. Thus, the CDM provides compelling evidence that the divide among Americans can be bridged enough to reach agreement on some desirable actions.

The CDM is fundamentally a problem-solving, trust-building methodology with easily recognizable and achievable steps that could be replicated in other geographic areas served by public health. Thus, for any organizations such as state and local health departments or community-based organizations that have authority and responsibility for making public health–related policy decisions, and in the multiple topic areas where competing values are at stake in making those decisions, CDM could be employed. Such topic areas include decisions about the use of nonpharmaceutical interventions during outbreaks or in a pandemic, policy choices aiming at violence prevention and gun control, vaccination policy issues, choices about access to abortion and other medical services, options for improved control of obesity, harm-reduction strategies related to drug addiction and recovery, and many others. Use of CDM in these types of situations could serve to trigger greater use of public participation in public health policymaking overall.

With additional recruiting and design modifications, the model could be scaled up to help bring a larger, unified voice of the public in any given area to the public health policymaking table.[7] Such inclusion of the public has the potential to be a trust-building and transformative strategy for public health. Greater public participation promotes some of the same concepts and principles underlying shared decision-making in clinical practice.[8] In that setting, the provider and patient collaborate to make the best-informed

AJPH October 2023, Vol 113, No. 10

decisions aligned with the patient's values. Just as in clinical settings where the goal is a more patient-centered care, the goal for public participation in community settings would be a more population-centered public health where sound decisions are well-aligned with public values. AJPH

ABOUT THE AUTHOR

Roger H. Bernier is an epidemiologist in Aiken, SC.

CORRESPONDENCE

Correspondence should be sent to Roger H. Bernier, 153 Crescent Point, Aiken, SC 29803 (e-mail: rogbernier@gmail.com). Reprints can be ordered at https://ajph.org by clicking the "Reprints" link.

PUBLICATION INFORMATION

Full Citation: Bernier RH. The Crosscurrents Dialogue Model: 2019–2023. *Am J Public Health*. 2023;113(10):1099–1101.

Acceptance Date: May 25, 2023.

DOI: https://doi.org/10.2105/AJPH.2023.307359

ACKNOWLEDGMENTS

I wish to thank the approximately 50 South Carolina citizens who participated in one or more of the 12 dialogues that were held on 10 separate topics since 2019. Especially, I wish to thank the current dialoguers from across the political spectrum, many of whom have been engaged for multiple years.

CONFLICTS OF INTEREST

There are no conflicts of interest to declare. No outside funding was used for this work.

HUMAN PARTICIPANT PROTECTION

Human participant protection is not applicable. This practice activity is a case example of dialogue methods and conversations used voluntarily by individuals to reach agreements among themselves on public issues.

REFERENCES

1. Galea S. Debating tradeoffs, sharing ideas. October 22, 2022. Available at: https://sandrogalea.substack.com/p/debating-tradeoffs-sharing-ideas?utm_source=%2Fsearch%2Fpublic%2520health%2520is%2520politics&utm_medium=reader2. Accessed May 26, 2023.
2. Boyle P. Public problems, values, and choices. School of Government University of North Carolina. 2001. Available at: https://www.sog.unc.edu/sites/default/files/articles/article3_8.pdf. Accessed May 26, 2023.
3. Commonwealth Fund. Meeting America's public health challenge. June 21, 2022. Available at: https://www.commonwealthfund.org/publications/fund-reports/2022/jun/meeting-americas-public-health-challenge. Accessed May 26, 2023.
4. DeSalvo K, Hughes B, Bassett M, et al. Public health COVID-19 impact assessment: lessons learned and compelling needs. National Academy of Medicine. April 7, 2021. Available at: https://nam.edu/public-health-covid-19-impact-assessment-lessons-learned-and-compelling-needs. Accessed May 26, 2023.
5. Osher Lifelong Learning Institute, University of South Carolina Beaufort. Curriculum guide. Winter/Spring 2023. Available at: https://www.uscb.edu/lifelong-learning/olli/pdfs/WinterSpring%202023%20Curriculum%20Guide_Online.pdf. Accessed May 26, 2023.
6. Montlake S. In Ohio, one man's quest to get more voters to agree to disagree. November 10, 2022. *Christian Science Monitor*. Available at: https://www.csmonitor.com/USA/Politics/2022/1110/In-Ohio-one-man-s-quest-to-get-more-voters-to-agree-to-disagree. Accessed May 26, 2023.
7. Bernier RH. Lessons learned from implementing a multi-year, multi-project public engagement initiative to better inform governmental public health policy decisions. *Participat Med*. 2014;6:e8. Available at: https://participatorymedicine.org/journal/evidence/case-studies/2014/05/22/lessons-learned-from-implementing-a-multi-year-multi-project-public-engagement-initiative-to-better-inform-governmental-public-health-policy-decisions/. Accessed May 26, 2023.
8. Elwyn G, Frosch D, Thomson R, et al. Shared decision-making: a model for clinical practice. *J Gen Intern Med*. 2012;27(10):1361–1367. https://doi.org/10.1007/s11606-012-2077-6

Overcoming Public Health "Surveillance": When Words Matter

William J. Kassler, MD, MPH, and Courtney L. Bowman, BA, BS

ABOUT THE AUTHORS

William Kassler was with Palantir Technologies, Denver, CO, during preparation of the article. Courtney Bowman is with Palantir Technologies.

See also Building Common Ground, pp. 1093–1115.

Public health surveillance is undertaken to inform both disease prevention and control. Defined as "the continuous, systematic collection, analysis and interpretation of health-related data needed for the planning, implementation, and evaluation of public health practice," surveillance underlies the myriad critical activities of a health department, from early detection to intervention and evaluation.[1(p14)] We would be hard pressed to look at our modern understanding of disease without attributing much of that knowledge to past surveillance. It is also hard to imagine how public health agencies would respond to an emerging infectious disease outbreak or design effective programs for noncommunicable disease without the situational awareness that comes from our surveillance systems.

The term itself is derived from the French roots *sur* (over) and *veiller* (to watch) and is defined in the dictionary as the "close and continuous observation of one or more persons for the purpose of direction, supervision, or control."[2] To public health professionals, that sounds like the practice of epidemiology, but for most people, the term has connotations that are quite different from public health. Most people associate surveillance with being watched over by ever-present security cameras and law enforcement staking out suspects. More recently, the term surveillance capitalism or surveillance for profit has been applied to big tech's role in data collection, creating social media algorithms, and spying on its end users to target ads and influence consumer behaviors.[3] In authoritarian countries, surveillance can take on a more sinister connotation of state social control of its population using increasingly sophisticated tools to both track and coerce more "socially acceptable" behaviors.[4]

Traditionally, public health surveillance has focused on using deidentified data to track patterns of risk factors and disease within populations, which is markedly different from tracking and controlling individuals. However, recent developments in technology, and the amount of personally identified information being collected via the Web, apps, and devices, accelerated by the use of electronic exposure notification for the COVID-19 pandemic, have further blurred those lines in perception if not in practice and have contributed to the erosion of the public's trust in governmental institutions.

BACKLASH

Historically, public health surveillance has not been without controversy. Named HIV reporting, for example, received substantial backlash due to its potential to expose marginalized populations to stigma and potential discrimination. However, concerns about surveillance seemed to have grown during the pandemic. This is in part because of the intense politicization of disease control, but also in part because of the scale and scope of these activities (COVID-19 illness, restrictions, and economic effects touched nearly everyone), aided in no small part by data proliferation and novel technologies.

Surveillance for COVID-19 used a combination of anonymized health data, nonanonymized clinical information, and other sources of data to track population-level patterns of disease and risk factors. These were often linked in the public's mind with disease control interventions that tracked individuals such as app- and device-based contact tracing and exposure notification.

Traditional contact tracing typically involves in-person interviews and a relationship of trust between the interviewer and the interviewee with the intent of understanding their movements and notifying individuals at risk for infection to get tested and, if indicated, preemptively self-quarantine.[5] Electronic device–based contact tracing and exposure notification, by contrast, were envisioned as a technology-facilitated version of the traditional technique that—wittingly or unwittingly—traded the virtues of a trust-dependent interpersonal interaction with the scalable capacity to track users' precise location in real time—where they are, where they have been, and whom they have consorted with. The idea was that—in its decentralized permutation—individuals could be alerted of their potential exposure and take appropriate measures or—in its centralized models—officials could then use those data to identify individuals who had been exposed and those who might infect others, potentially linking that information to isolation or quarantine orders. Adding to the confusion, digital vaccine passports and symptom trackers, also based on smartphone apps, were explicitly linked to people's ability to work, travel, and access public spaces.

Furthermore, because many state public health departments did not have the resources or know-how to build complex platforms, many agencies outsourced traditional state-based public health surveillance to tech companies. In some cases, tech companies took it upon themselves to engineer solutions unprompted by the government agencies formally charged with these duties.[6] This drive toward technology "solutionism" and industry intervention[7] has only served to further erode trust from a public that already has grown weary of corporate priorities that emphasize the unfettered monetization of the data.

The resulting pushback on the exercise of the police powers of public health points to an urgent need to reframe epidemiological surveillance.

WORDS MATTER

At a time when our beliefs and values are deeply constituted and reinforced as partisan ideologies, the way we interpret information and use it to form opinions is filtered through distinctly different and polarized lenses. Widely established consensus, such as the value of immunization or other scientific approaches to public health, appear to be weakening. Even the most seemingly inoffensive terms such as "security" or "education" can be laden with meaning, often with political overtones. One of the most surprising outcomes of the pandemic is the extent to which many Americans seemed to fuse their political ideology to rejection of science-based interventions and core public health practices. This resulted in widespread distrust of public health institutions.

In 2017, the Robert Wood Johnson Foundation published the results of an extensive multimodal initiative using survey and market research to find a common language around health issues—specifically, to identify how people with different political perspectives understand health issues, how different messages were received by political segments, and what types of messages resonate across the spectrum.[8] An effective message cannot be politically loaded, avoids hot buttons, does not evoke either conscious or unconscious negative reactions, preferably includes values from both conservatives and progressives, and is not overly academic. That is a tall order.

One optimistic sign comes from North Carolina. A group of payers, providers, and community-based organizations commissioned Democratic and Republican polling firms to conduct a series of focus groups to learn how people think and talk about health.[9] They found considerable agreement spanning the economic, political, racial, and rural–urban divides on housing, food insecurity, and living wages, and even on allocating resources between health care and community. However, they also observed that the terms used by public health to describe these issues were confusing, alienating, and demeaning, and served to obscure rather than bridge shared values.

In linguistics, the notion of reclamation is used to describe the cultural process through which words that have been sullied by pejorative associations are rehabilitated to restore an earlier, less-fraught intent.[10] Restoring "surveillance" to represent in the public eye a more virtuous public health focus unencumbered by the pervasive connotations of control, threat detection, policing, and manipulation may, however, be a bridge too far. The phrase has become saddled with a focus on ubiquitous and intrusive personal oversight for the purposes of mastery, exploitation, or worse. For an epidemiological practice that, instead, regards the individual as a source to be carefully guarded and whose data matter most as an aggregated indicator of the effect of contagious pathogens on public health at large, "surveillance" may be a phrase beyond rehabilitation. Indeed, there is a time for reclamation and a time for cutting losses and adopting a fresh approach to talking about an essential practice of public health.

To cut loose public health from an increasingly stigmatized association and rebuild trust in our public health institutions grounded in a values orientation that transcends partisan lines, we call on the field to reframe surveillance. Turning away from ocular metaphors (i.e., expressions that evoke watching, seeing, supervision, and the like) might be an important step to shaking off the residual discomfiture. Perhaps a metaphor like public health's radar or an explanatory phrase such as situational awareness will resonate. Effective messaging will also require social marketing and communications expertise and an initiative to develop and test the frame. It will require attention and discipline to ensure that the new framing is not cynically received as a marketing exploit to cover problems that persist under the surface.

SURVEILLANCE AND TECHNOLOGY

Beyond acknowledging that our language might not be serving us well, we must therefore also acknowledge and address the underlying threats of technology-based surveillance on public health practices. Going forward, these new surveillance modalities are likely to persist and expand. Data modernization is a multimillion-dollar program to invest in new data sources and new information systems to improve public health surveillance and response. New data, arising from the digital footprints of our online presence, search logs, and social media feeds, and the geocoded and biometric data streaming from our wearable sensors (e.g., Fitbits, smart watches, fitness apps) can all be rich sources of behavioral and health status information. These novel data sources, combined with clinical data aggregated at scale from electronic health records and advances in analytics such as machine learning, offer real promise to transform public health.[11] But they are not without risk. The more data sources that can be combined, the easier it becomes to reidentify anonymized individuals, and the greater potential for reconstructive identification that bad government actors and for-profit data miners can use to create detailed profiles of individuals. In the wrong hands, this information has the potential to compromise privacy, cause individual harm, and exacerbate health inequities. Modern forms of surveillance have morphed into something John Snow, the father of epidemiology, would not recognize and represent much more of a threat to civil liberties.

PRIVACY AS A UNITING THEME

While people with different political perspectives see the world differently, both progressives and conservatives share common concerns about the right to privacy.[12,13] Though the word "privacy" does not appear explicitly in the US Constitution, there are few liberties more universally American than the "right to be let alone."[14(p221)] More formally enshrined guarantees against unwanted intrusions of speech and assembly (1st Amendment), protection against unwarranted search and seizure of personal property and effects (4th Amendment), equal protection under the law; limitations on state depravations of life, liberty, and property; and guarantees of due process (14th Amendment) all remain steadfast touchpoints for citizens across the political spectrum.

At a moment in American history of seemingly unprecedented political division and limited opportunities for bipartisanship, privacy is indeed one of the few issues over which both sides of the aisle are willing to bridge their differences. In its last session, Congress came closer than it has in decades to comprehensive consumer privacy reform with the American Data Privacy and Protection Act, agreeing largely in principle with the broader legislative contours, but stalling on lingering concerns about federal preemption and private right of action. More critically, legislative action reflects constituent concern, with poll after poll suggesting that the majority of Americans want stronger protections over their personal information.[12]

Even while public trust in bedrock public sector institutions may be at its nadir, there is an unparalleled opportunity to leverage privacy as a rare unifying concern that has also captured a sizable share of the public's attention.

BEYOND WORDS

Whether public health surveillance is ultimately reframed, it is clear that the epidemiological regime to come will need to establish protecting data privacy and restoring public trust as foremost objectives. This will be no mean task, given the temptation to continue to draw upon many of the same technologies otherwise fueling the surveillance capitalism data economy: smart devices, ubiquitous sensors, advertising technology, and data proliferation.

The good news is that many of the principles, tools, and frameworks for responsible use of sensitive information are well-established and work. What is needed, however, in modernizing public health "surveillance" is a redoubled focus on these elements and a comprehensive view of how they all fit together to foster an ecosystem of accountability and trust.

Central to this proposed shift is the elevation of the privacy by design and by default cultural paradigm.[15] This means that the standard configuration of technologies used for public health applications must be developed and deployed to achieve a maximally privacy-protective state, rather than in a configuration that exclusively preferences data utility, speed, cost, or other optimization considerations.

A privacy by design and by default technology approach further entails the following use of trusted privacy-enhancing technologies including capabilities that provide that

- personal data are accessed and shared according to explicit and deliberate patient consent and permission by the responsible organization or entity;
- data permissioning is granular and flexible enough to be modified over time as risk profiles, consent, and use agreements are modified to expand or contract data access and use;

- data processing and analysis supports a broad range of de-identification techniques, including generalization, aggregation, obfuscation on demand, obfuscation by default, dynamic minimization, and statistical anonymization;
- information systems used to carry out public health functions include robust auditing capabilities that empower oversight bodies to check and verify compliance with data governance policies and investigate potential misuses;
- systems support the ability to test and validate data before they are applied to consequential outcomes or are shared more widely;
- comprehensive data lineage tracing, including transparency into how data flow through a data ecosystem, is enabled; and
- personal data are deleted by default once their retention is no longer justified or consented to.

This set of desiderata is indicative, not necessarily exhaustive. But, even beyond privacy by design and by default cultural best practices and practical utilization of privacy-enhancing technologies, regaining public trust in the use of these technologies will require commensurate investment in institutional governance and communications. Ethics guidelines should be administered by designated and appropriately resourced bodies. These bodies should be endowed with the teeth to invoke censure and revoke data access when ethical principles and privacy requirements are transgressed. Similarly, the details of technology protections and program governance should be proactively and continuously communicated—and at a meaningful and accessible register for public consumption—to community members, especially those most vulnerable to the impacts of such programs.

CONCLUSION

Decades of chronic underfunding have left our public health infrastructure frayed, and the pandemic exposed the critical weaknesses within our federal, state, and local health systems.[16] With our deep, pervasive, and evenly divided electorate, few opportunities exist to bridge these gaps. Yet, bipartisan support from appropriators and policymakers is needed to secure the level of investment necessary to strengthen and modernize our data and information systems toward a common goal of health. A critical step toward achieving this support is to reframe surveillance in a way that resonates across the aisle, and to assure that the programs and systems we develop emphasize the same high priority for privacy and civil liberties that our policymakers and their constituents demand. AJPH

CORRESPONDENCE

Correspondence should be sent to William Kassler, MD, MPH, Palantir Technologies, 1200 17th St, Floor 15, Denver, CO 80202 (e-mail: wkassler@gmail.com). Reprints can be ordered at https://ajph.org by clicking the "Reprints" link.

PUBLICATION INFORMATION

Full Citation: Kassler WJ, Bowman CL. Overcoming public health "surveillance": when words matter. *Am J Public Health*. 2023;113(10):1102–1105.

Acceptance Date: May 19, 2023.

DOI: https://doi.org/10.2105/AJPH.2023.307348

CONTRIBUTORS

Both authors certify that they have contributed substantially to the concept, drafting and revision of the article, and the approval of the final version.

CONFLICTS OF INTEREST

During the preparation of this article, both authors were employed by Palantir Technologies, a software engineering firm that develops and sells information systems to public health agencies.

REFERENCES

1. WHO guidelines on ethical issues in public health surveillance. Geneva, Switzerland: World Health Organization; 2017. Available at: https://apps.who.int/iris/bitstream/handle/10665/255721/9789241512657-eng.pdf. Accessed February 5, 2023.
2. Choi BCK. The past, present, and future of public health surveillance. *Scientifica (Cairo)*. 2012;2012:875253. https://doi.org/10.6064/2012/875253
3. Zuboff S, Schwandt K. *The Age of Surveillance Capitalism: The Fight for a Human Future at the New Frontier of Power*. New York, NY: PublicAffairs; 2019.
4. Lyon D. *Pandemic Surveillance*. Cambridge, MA: Polity Press; 2022.
5. Langmuir AD. The surveillance of communicable diseases of national importance. *N Engl J Med*. 1963;268(4):182–192. https://doi.org/10.1056/NEJM196301242680405
6. Apple and Google partner on COVID-19 contact tracing technology. Apple Newsroom. April 10, 2020. Available at: https://www.apple.com/newsroom/2020/04/apple-and-google-partner-on-covid-19-contact-tracing-technology. Accessed February 5, 2023.
7. Morozov E. *To Save Everything, Click Here: The Folly of Technological Solutionism*. New York, NY: PublicAffairs; 2013.
8. Carger E, Westen D. A new way to talk about the social determinants of health. Robert Wood Johnson Foundation. January 1, 2010. Available at: https://www.rwjf.org/en/library/research/2010/01/a-new-way-to-talk-about-the-social-determinants-of-health.html. Accessed February 5, 2023.
9. Lumpkin JR, Perla R, Onie R, Seligson R. What we need to be healthy—and how to talk about it. *Health Affairs Forefront*. May 3, 2021. Available at: https://www.healthaffairs.org/do/10.1377/forefront.20210429.335599. Accessed February 5, 2023.
10. Coles G. The exorcism of language: reclaimed derogatory terms and their limits. *College English*. 2016;78(5):424–446. Available at: https://www.jstor.org/stable/44075135. Accessed February 5, 2023.
11. Kassler WJ. Public health informatics, big data, advanced analytics, and emerging technology. In: Fraser MR, Castrucci BC, eds. *Building Strategic Skills for Better Health: A Primer for Public Health Professionals*. New York, NY: Oxford University Press; 2023.
12. Weust J. A conservative right to privacy: legal, ideological, and coalitional transformations in US social conservatism. *Law Soc Inquiry*. 2021;46(4):964–992. https://doi.org/10.1017/lsi.2021.1
13. Godlasky A. American Data Privacy and Protection Act (ADPPA) didn't pass but got further than ever. National Press Foundation. November 30, 2022. Available at: https://nationalpress.org/topic/data-privacy-act-adppa-us-lacks-law-eu-standard. Accessed February 5, 2023.
14. Brandeis LD, Warren SD. The right to privacy. *Harv Law Rev*. 1890;4:221.
15. Cavoukian A. Privacy by design: the 7 foundational principles. 2011. Available at: https://iapp.org/media/pdf/resource_center/pbd_implement_7found_principles.pdf. Accessed July 18, 2023.
16. The impact of chronic underfunding on America's public health system: trends, risks, and recommendations, 2022. Trust for America's Health. Available at: https://www.tfah.org/wp-content/uploads/2022/07/2022PublicHealthFundingFINAL.pdf. Accessed February 5, 2023.

I Hear You: Seeking Population Health Common Ground

Sanne Magnan, MD, PhD, and David Kindig, MD, PhD

ABOUT THE AUTHORS

Sanne Magnan is with the HealthPartners Institute, Bloomington, MN. David Kindig is with the University of Wisconsin–Madison School of Medicine and Public Health, Madison.

See also Building Common Ground, pp. 1093–1115.

Listening for common ground requires suspension of assumptions and openness to diverse ideas. One of us (D. K.) wrote in 2015: "I refuse to join, however, with many people on both the left and the right of the political spectrum who claim that the same ideological differences that poison our efforts on hot-button issues . . . also must block efforts to improve population health."[1(p24)] Although written eight years ago in the article "Can There Be Political Common Ground for Improving Population Health?" the state of political and ideological differences in America (and indeed the world) has reached greater levels that threaten progress in many domains. It is one thing to "refuse to join"; it is another to achieve meaningful common ground. Savage articulates principles of building common ground from "frustration to friendship" in an individual office.[2] In a different vein, *AJPH* is providing needed leadership to explore the opportunities and challenges for building common ground in public health and population health policy.

What is common ground? It occurs when two people or groups "agree about something, especially when they do not agree about other things" (https://bit.ly/3scCgzi). Easy to say, difficult to do. We list here a dozen principles or considerations that may be helpful in fostering such agreement in the field:

1. Start with understanding people as people—what is most important to them (e.g., values, families of origin,[3] and important milestones). Elicit narratives and life experiences that are "their ground." Look for things you have in common. For example, an elected Democrat, Jared Mead, and an elected Republican, Nate Nehring, on the Snohomish County Council in Washington State recently began hosting events in their community—"Building Bridges"—for meaningful dialogue. "After we all shared a bit about our family histories and where our kids are going to school, it naturally became much more difficult to demonize one another." These two politicians believe that ". . . being open to honest conversations on tough subjects can go a long way in arriving at common ground," and they have worked together on public health issues such as housing, the environment, and early childhood education.[4]
2. Act with good intentions. Listen without judgment to different viewpoints. Engage with curiosity, ask honest questions, and be humble.[3,5] At the 2022 American Public Health Association Annual Meeting opening session, Loretta J. Ross said, "call in" people versus "call out" in an aggressive hostile manner as we have seen in our public sphere. "Calling in is holding people accountable, but you use love and respect, not because of who they are, but because of who you are. Love and respect needs to be our public health strategy."[6] Through the Center for Prevention and Study of Violence, part of the Institute of Behavioral Science at the University of Colorado Boulder, the Gun Shop Project (in other states as well) calls in gun shop retailers in the fight against suicides with education and resources. Framing, messaging, trust, and honesty are critically important for this common ground. With a Centers for Disease Control and Prevention grant, University of Colorado Boulder researchers are evaluating the project.[7,8]
3. Create safe places to discuss perspectives. One approach is "public deliberation" when the issues are complex, and understanding perspective disagreements among the public is valuable to health policymakers.[9] Researchers, for example when using public deliberation during the early stages of COVID-19 vaccinations, noted that "These circumstances commonly involve priority setting for programs and initiatives where resources are scarce and there are competing

AJPH October 2023, Vol 113, No. 10

values and obligations."[10(p87)] Erika Blacksher and colleagues, with funding from County Health Rankings and Roadmaps, a program of the Robert Wood Johnson Foundation, are exploring the creation of a toolkit for deliberative dialogue and decision-making. Can structured dialogue "disrupt everyday reasoning habits, short-circuit stereotypes, and cultivate population health dialogues that are more curious, inclusive, and characterized by mutual concern and trust" (https://bit.ly/3OMWHMj)?

4. "Exit the echo chamber."[5(p158)] In the chapter with this title in *I Think You're Wrong (But I'm Listening)*, Holland and Silvers describe actions to challenge confirmation bias. For example, read three articles from news sources that are not your typical source. Go to coffee with someone and explore how and why they voted differently. Draw an "empathy map" for someone in another political party (e.g., What do they think and feel? What do they hear? What do they see? What do they say and do? What pain and needs do they have?[5[p171]]). "Empathy does not equal endorsement"[5(p113)]; it is for understanding the other side and for better understanding ourselves.
5. Do not describe solutions as an initial step. Rachel Block from Milbank Memorial Fund in a conversation (January 4, 2023) recommends to first create a common way to describe a problem. Faithful Families Thriving Communities (Faithful Families; https://faithfulfamilies.com), initially a partnership for faith-based communities between the North Carolina Division of Public Health and North Carolina State Extension, focused on obesity but quickly learned to listen to the priorities of faith communities and understand their perspectives and assets—not just seeing these communities as dissemination points for health promotion. Over time, the initiative grew the capacity of lay leaders to address health policies and disparities with more local and national partnerships across public health, practitioners, and researchers. Faithful Families works to share power through a collaborative process of including others in decisions that affect the program. Going forward, a significant challenge is sustaining this engagement beyond a "program" implementation.[11]
6. Understand the moral foundations of opponents to your policy proposal. Jonathan Haidt identifies that while both liberals and conservatives share values like caring, liberty, and fairness, conservatives also tend to embrace others like loyalty, authority, and sanctity,[12] and says this breadth is a conservative advantage. Public health, which is typically liberal leaning, can expand its approach to achieve public health goals. An example is the North Carolina Harm Reduction Coalition advocating for a needle exchange program in the devastating opioid and heroin epidemic. The Coalition worked with public health, the substance abuse recovery community, legislators, medical professionals, law enforcement, and others to create a moral foundation that would resonate in this politically divided state. "Conservative lawmakers were able to adhere to their traditional stance of being tough on crime and of having an aversion to degradation of the human body, both significant moral foundations in conservative communities. The advocacy process focused on preserving the values of sound economics, respect for law (*Authority*), and moral traditions of compassion for families within their communities (*Care, Loyalty, and Sanctity*)."[13(p422)] Subsequently, a 2016 authorization for sterile needle exchange programs was created in North Carolina.[13]
7. Explore messaging for your proposal that addresses others' values, even if you are not likely to change these core values or moral foundations. Gollust et al. show that messages highlighting the negative impact of childhood obesity on military readiness "increased conservatives' perceptions that nonindividual actors (the government, food and beverage companies, and schools) bear responsibility for addressing obesity, and increased their support for policy action."[14(p.e101)] However, the authors caution that novel messages should be tested to avoid backlash or further stigmatization in this case of obese individuals.
8. Carefully consider the fairness foundation when addressing equity. Haidt argues that fairness is shared by both political ideologies, but he points out a nuance about this value domain: "Everyone cares about fairness, but there are two major kinds. On the left, fairness often implies equality, but on the right it means

proportionality—people should be rewarded in proportion to what they contribute, even if that guarantees unequal outcomes."[12(p160–161)] Finding common ground or at the least recognizing the ideological differences regarding fairness may be one of the toughest challenges in improving health equity. A recent example is a major issue in the debt ceiling talks regarding work requirements for certain Supplemental Nutrition Assistance Program recipients. Common ground was found when Republicans proposed increasing the age requirement, but Democrats responded by exempting veterans and homeless persons, allowing the overall bill to progress.

However, this common ground will leave some persons without benefits. As Jones points out, "For the people directly affected, the culture war is a real war too. They know there is no safety in the in-between. The romance of the middle can exist when one's empathy is aligned with the people expressing opinions on policy or culture rather than with those who will be affected by these policies or cultural norms" (https://bit.ly/3YADoZR).

9. Explore opportunities in crises to build common ground. For example, although the Dakota Access Pipeline strained relationships between North Dakota and the Standing Rock Sioux Tribe, both sides in 2020 were worried about the emerging coronavirus. North Dakota state, North Dakota Department of Health, and the tribe through the North Dakota Indian Commission worked together on mobile testing on the reservation.[15] Messages from joint trusted sources of the North Dakota Indian Commission and the University of North Dakota School of Medicine and Health Sciences provided clear public health approaches for tribes.[16] One former North Dakota health official (M. Tufte, e-mail communication, May 26, 2023) said this work was healing for relationships.
10. Look for uncommon allies. The Colorado School of Public Health hosted a candid panel in 2023 on "National Security and the Impact on Public Health" with military leaders to explore national security issues and threats, especially political extremism ". . . which certainly spill over into public health—in obvious and sometimes not so obvious ways." Protecting our communities from diseases such as COVID-19 can intersect with strategies to protect against "political and ideological contagions that threaten the social fabric." One panel member said, "We want to take the sense of meaning that individuals may find in extremism and put it back into something positive." Public health assessments and best practices are ways to interact and support veterans in a holistic manner—especially those who struggle after leaving the military. With allies of the military and the Veterans Administration, the three areas of public health to address are prevention, education, and rehabilitation. Another topic discussed was assisting refugee communities and the distinct roles of the military and public health. A Canadian military official highlighted the benefits of finding the intersection of national security and public health: "Great minds don't think alike . . . They challenge each other to think again."[17]
11. Identify the power player(s) and what is important to them. Who leads on the issue, what is needed for their perseverance, and what are the underlying power dynamics that impact the final common ground according to former public health nurse, now–North Carolina Senator Gale Adcock (D-NC; oral and e-mail communication, May 30 and June 6, 2023)? For example, North Carolina Governor Roy Cooper (D-NC) kept Medicaid expansion "on the table," (Gale Adcock; oral and e-mail communication, May 30 and June 6, 2023) vetoing the 2019–2020 budget bill that did not include expansion. North Carolina Senate President Pro-Tempore Phil Berger (R-NC), who had long opposed Medicaid expansion, signaled a change in his perspective in 2022 because of these factors: the federal government not reneging (over the previous decade) on its commitment to cover 90% of expansion costs, North Carolina's ability to fund the other 10% through assessments on hospitals and Medicaid managed care companies, the change from fee-for-service to more cost-predictable managed care, rural hospital closures and financial instability, and public support for expansion. A "sign-on" bonus from the federal government of approximately 1.8 billion dollars was an economic tipping point. To bring his colleagues and constituents along, Senator Berger publicly explained how his thinking had evolved.[18–20]

12. Expect discomfort but do not create disdain or contempt.[3] Getting outside of your comfort zone will be uncomfortable; however, being challenged will sharpen skills and increase awareness of how to relate to others with different perspectives. Nonetheless, if the situation becomes toxic and traumatizing, there is a time to walk away.[3,21]

These principles and considerations, however, are not a recipe for success, and there may be others to add. Nonetheless, there is some caution about serious risks across polarized divides—Read lists three: "(1) masking important differences between oneself and a polarized opponent, thereby inhibiting efforts to respond appropriately to such differences; (2) submitting oneself to undue (physical, cognitive, and emotional) harms; and (3) exacerbating intergroup hostility and antagonism when finding common ground across one group divide negatively highlights differences across another." She does say in some circumstances that there can be value in exploring common ground, which may mitigate harmful relationships by surfacing points of shared concern or common goals, even if the initial disagreement discussion does not lead to common ground (https://bit.ly/4415PRN). The opinion editorial "The Potential and Challenges for Common Ground on Abortion" by one of us (S. M.) explores such an approach with disagreements (https://bit.ly/443tlh7).

Despite these warnings, the intolerance building in our society is not a good recipe for a democracy, particularly as evident on college campuses and recently in the House of Representatives. However, for leaders in public health and population health, these 12 principles or considerations, and the other ideas in this issue, may help produce meaningful and substantial common ground in the coming decade. AJPH

CORRESPONDENCE

Correspondence should be sent to Sanne Magnan, HealthPartners Institute, Mailstop 21112R, PO Box 1309, Minneapolis, MN 55440-1309 (e-mail: sannemagnan@gmail.com). Reprints can be ordered at https://ajph.org by clicking the "Reprints" link.

PUBLICATION INFORMATION

Full Citation: Magnan S, Kindig D. I hear you: seeking population health common ground. *Am J Public Health.* 2023;113(10):1106–1109.

Acceptance Date: June 23, 2023.

DOI: https://doi.org/10.2105/AJPH.2023.307373

CONTRIBUTORS

S. Magnan and D. Kindig both contributed to the conceptualization, design, writing, and editing of the article.

CONFLICTS OF INTEREST

The authors report no conflicts of interest.

REFERENCES

1. Kindig DA. Can there be political common ground for improving population health? *Milbank Q.* 2015;93(1):24–27. https://doi.org/10.1111/1468-0009.12101
2. Savage S. From frustration to friend: how building common ground made us better. Thin Difference. June 15, 2017. Available at: https://www.thindifference.com/2017/06/building-common-ground-made-us-better. Accessed June 8, 2023.
3. Holland SS, Silvers B. *Now What? How to Move Forward When We're Divided (About Basically Everything).* Grand Rapids, MI: Revell; 2022.
4. Mead J, Nehring N. We are proof that Democrats and Republicans can work together. *Seattle Times.* February 28, 2023. Available at: https://www.seattletimes.com/opinion/we-are-proof-that-democrats-and-republicans-can-work-together. Accessed June 5, 2023.
5. Holland SS, Silvers B. *I Think You're Wrong (But I'm Listening)—A Guide to Grace-Filled Political Conversations.* Nashville, TN: Nelson Books; 2019.
6. Barna M. Opening general session: "Love and respect needs to be our public health strategy." Public Health Newswire. November 6, 2022. Available at: http://www.publichealthnewswire.org/?p=opening_general_session_2022. Accessed June 5, 2023.
7. Marshall L. Why working with gun retailers is critical in the fight against suicides. *CU Boulder Today.* March 4, 2021. Available at: https://www.colorado.edu/today/2021/03/04/why-working-gun-retailers-critical-fight-against-suicide. Accessed June 6, 2023.
8. Polzer E, Brandspigel S, Kelly T, Betz M. "Gun shop projects" for suicide prevention in the USA: current state and future directions. *Inj Prev.* 2021;27(2):150–154. https://doi.org/10.1136/injuryprev-2020-043648
9. Degeling C, Carter SM, Rychetnik L. Which public and why deliberate?—a scoping review of public deliberation in public health and health policy research. *Soc Sci Med.* 2015;131:114–121. https://doi.org/10.1016/j.socscimed.2015.03.009
10. Scherer M, Kamler A, Weiss L, Blacksher E, Jeavons J, Gold M. Using public deliberation to set priorities: the case of COVID-19 vaccine access in New York City. *J Public Health Manag Pract.* 2022;28(1):86–94. https://doi.org/10.1097/PHH.0000000000001471
11. Hardison-Moody A, Yao J. Faithful families, thriving communities: bridging faith and health through a state-level partnership. *Am J Public Health.* 2019;109(3):363–368. https://doi.org/10.2105/AJPH.2018.304869
12. Haidt J. *The Righteous Mind: Why Good People Are Divided by Politics and Religion.* New York, NY: Vintage Books; 2013.
13. Matthews G, Burris S, Ledford SL, Gunderson G, Baker EL. Crafting richer public health messages for a turbulent political environment. *J Public Health Manag Pract.* 2017;23(4):420–423. https://doi.org/10.1097/PHH.0000000000000610
14. Gollust SE, Niederdeppe J, Barry CL. Framing the consequences of childhood obesity to increase public support for obesity prevention policy. *Am J Public Health.* 2013;103(11):e96–e102. https://doi.org/10.2105/AJPH.2013.301271
15. Benth M. Native American reservations could see another round of COVID-19 testing. *KFYR TV.* May 28, 2020. Available at: https://www.kfyrtv.com/content/news/Native-American-reservations-could-see-another-round-of-COVID-19-testing-570850291.html. Accessed June 8, 2023.
16. Warne D. COVID-19 tribal information—"Have Compassion" video. Available at: https://www.indianaffairs.nd.gov/initiatives/healthcare/covid-19-tribal-information. Accessed June 8, 2023.
17. Colorado School of Public Health. National security and public health find common ground in panel discussion. March 7, 2023. Available at: https://coloradosph.cuanschutz.edu/research-and-practice/practice/public-health-main-site-news/national-security-and-public-health-find-common-ground-in-panel-discussion. Accessed June 7, 2023.
18. Searing A. Why North Carolina is finally getting to "yes" on Medicaid expansion. Georgetown University Health Policy Institute. March 10, 2023. Available at: https://ccf.georgetown.edu/2023/03/10/why-north-carolina-is-finally-saying-yes-to-medicaid-expansion. Accessed May 31, 2023.
19. Akin S. How N.C. got to yes on Medicaid expansion. *Pluribus News.* April 4, 2023. Available at: https://pluribusnews.com/news-and-events/how-n-c-got-to-yes-on-medicaid-expansion. Accessed May 31, 2023.
20. Governor Cooper signs Medicaid expansion into law. NC Governor Roy Cooper. March 27, 2023. Available at: https://governor.nc.gov/news/press-releases/2023/03/27/governor-cooper-signs-medicaid-expansion-law. Accessed May 31, 2023.
21. Bennett J. What if instead of calling people out, we called them in? *New York Times.* November 19, 2020. Available at: https://www.nytimes.com/2020/11/19/style/loretta-ross-smith-college-cancel-culture.html. Accessed June 7, 2023.

Building a "We" With Deliberative Dialogue in Pursuit of Health for All

Erika Blacksher, PhD, Yukiko Asada, PhD, Marion Danis, MD, Marthe R. Gold, MD, MPH, Nellie Kassebaum, MPH, and Jarron Saint Onge, PhD

ABOUT THE AUTHORS

Erika Blacksher and Nellie Kassebaum are with the Center for Practical Bioethics, Kansas City, MO. Yukiko Asada and Marion Danis are with the Department of Bioethics, National Institutes of Health, Bethesda, MD. Marthe R. Gold is with CUNY School of Medicine, City College of New York, New York, NY. Jarron Saint Onge is with the Department of Population Health, School of Medicine, University of Kansas, Kansas City.

See also Building Common Ground, pp. 1093–1115.

Health in the United States is characterized by sizable inequalities by race, class, and geography; declining life expectancy; and a "health disadvantage" that makes the nation as a whole less healthy than other high-income countries.[1] Although explanations are multifactorial, numerous studies point upstream to federal and state policies that shape the social, economic, and environmental conditions in which people learn, live, work, play, and age.[1–4] Most Americans are unaware of these facts except as lived realities. We think they should have more meaningful opportunities to learn about and participate in policy decisions that affect their health and longevity.

Although citizens elect officials at state and federal levels to represent their policy preferences and values, voting is only one form of democracy, and often an imperfect one. Policy debate and the politics that shape it may lack credible evidence, be framed to persuade or incite, and reinforce stereotypes and "us" versus "them" narratives. For example, the politicization of COVID-19 vaccines and other mitigation measures generated significant disinformation, distrust, and resistance, helping to fuel the nation's outsized death toll.[5] But studies have also demonstrated that an association between deepening political divisions and state-level variations in health outcomes—life expectancy, infant mortality, and working-age mortality—predate the pandemic.[2–4] Made possible by shifts in power from the federal government to state governments over the last four decades, states have moved toward opposite ends of the political spectrum and remade policies on labor, welfare, guns, health care access, health behaviors (e.g., use of tobacco, marijuana), the environment, immigration, and civil rights, all of which affect residents' health.

A more deliberative democracy would offer a viable supplement to formal political processes of representation, better inform citizens, and serve as an antidote to the nation's polarizing policy and political discourse. In practice, deliberative democracy takes the form of "public deliberations" that convene people of varied backgrounds to learn and talk together about a social problem in search of solutions.[6] Studies have shown that participants gain knowledge, regardless of education level; get insight into others' lives and perspectives; develop trust in fellow participants and society; become more public spirited in reasoning and views; and exhibit less partisan animosity, even in deeply divided societies such as the United States.[7–14] We believe that deliberation designed and operationalized to address worrisome health trends has the potential to build a "we" in the pursuit of a healthier, more equitable nation.

CORE PRINCIPLES AND PRACTICES OF DELIBERATION

Over the last several decades, people working in policy, academic, and civic settings in the United States and around the world have developed models of deliberation to gather well-informed public input on tough value-laden questions for which there is no one right answer and about which people disagree. Although there are various methods of deliberation, they share core principles and practices.[6,15] First, deliberation requires diversity among participants. Meaningful diversity in perspectives can be achieved by recruiting people of varied social, racial, and educational backgrounds, abilities, ages, sexual orientations, genders, and political orientations. Because deliberation tends to attract people with more education, time, and money, organizers typically undertake intentional recruitment efforts to ensure that underserved groups and communities can participate.

Second, deliberations provide balanced information conveyed in plain language and framed for deliberation, not persuasion. Information about the relevant science comes from credible sources and addresses what is known and, where relevant, unknown. Information about varying philosophies or ethical opinions, if presented, encompasses a wide range of views.

Third, deliberations are value oriented. They pose questions that ask what should be done about an important social challenge. Participants are often asked to develop recommendations or set priorities. Facilitation probes for the reasons, beliefs, values, and experiences that underpin participants' views and priorities. The structure and facilitation of deliberation encourage careful weighing of evidence and a wide range of perspectives and underlying justifications.

Fourth, deliberations support inclusivity and equality among participants and the free exchange of ideas. The use of explicit ground rules and well-trained facilitators who actively moderate discussions can help achieve these ends. Welcoming diverse modes of communication, such as storytelling and testimony, and self-interest as a source of justification for one's views can broaden the range of beliefs, reasons, and values that become part of the discussion.

DELIBERATION IN HEALTH CARE AND PUBLIC HEALTH

Deliberations have been used in the United States and around the world to gather public input on social challenges in many social sectors, such as the environment, education, technology, transportation, and, increasingly, health care and public health.[16] Here are a few examples. Although dormant since 2015, the United Kingdom's National Institute for Health and Care Excellence established a standing citizen's council in 2002 to identify social values that should shape coverage decisions.[17] One issue addressed by the council was how to reduce health inequalities between social classes. A deliberative tool for setting health care priorities has been used in the United States and other countries and adapted to set priorities for public health, patient-centered health research, and the social determinants of health.[8] During the COVID-19 pandemic, online deliberations with diverse New Yorkers gathered views on how to distribute vaccines to essential workers.[18]

Yet, few deliberations have directly addressed the nation's worsening overall health and health inequalities by race, class, and geography.[19–21] What is known about public opinion on population health comes largely from surveys and focus groups, and their results suggest serious challenges to building broad public support for health-supportive policies. Not only are Americans relatively unaware that social and economic conditions influence human health, but some may reject such facts as biased or mistaken.[22,23] The frameworks and language of population health (e.g., "social determinants of health," "inequalities," "equity," "systems," "structural racism") can make some people uncomfortable, spark partisan tensions, and reduce support for upstream social solutions.[24,25] Some Americans may also react negatively to data sorted by social group categories (e.g., race, gender) and attribute blame for poor health based on biases about certain groups.[26]

These same studies also offer lessons for how to design deliberations that may open up discussion, rather than shut it down. First, information about how social arrangements affect everyone can garner the interest of Americans, regardless of political orientation.[23] Thus, information about the nation's overall poor health, which is most pronounced among minoritized and economically marginalized groups but also affects more advantaged Americans, may stimulate broad curiosity and openness to learning about upstream causes of health.

Second, information about trends over time versus specific incidents can help people think about structural influences on outcomes.[25] This finding suggests that information about the nation's overall poor health and health inequalities, which are population patterns that develop and change over time, may help balance the strong belief among many Americans that health outcomes are attributable primarily to individual choices and behaviors.[22]

Third, an inclusive account of the causes of health—from health behaviors to health care and social, economic, and environmental conditions—can reduce partisan responses to such information.[27] A broad account of health causation may even foster openness to social responsibility, because affirming something Americans generally do believe (i.e., individual behaviors cause health outcomes) may open people's minds to information they are less likely to believe (i.e., social and economic conditions cause health outcomes).[23]

A more difficult issue is how to present information about health inequalities between social groups. Such information is an essential element of inclusive and balanced information about US population health challenges, yet, as noted, such information may hamper discussion. However, presenting such information by multiple social groups (e.g., race, education, gender, rurality) may help differently situated Americans "see" themselves in health data. When possible, presenting health inequalities by multiple social groups simultaneously—or "intersectionally" (e.g., poor White women, poor Black women)—may also help convey the broad reach of poor health in America.

Racial concordance between experts and facilitators and participants has not, to our knowledge, been studied, but communication science supports the value of racial concordance between those who deliver and those who receive health information.[28] A racially diverse facilitation team and expert panel may help participants from all racial backgrounds feel comfortable sharing their stories in their own words.

OPERATIONALIZING DELIBERATION IN POPULATION HEALTH

Deliberation on questions of population health could have varied purposes at different levels of decision-making (e.g., local, state, federal). For example, at the community level, deliberation could inform the priorities of nonprofit hospital decisions about how best to meet community needs, health department decisions about strategic investments in community health, and extension services' efforts to address the needs of rural communities. These entities already do community outreach, needs assessments, and "deliberation-like" activities, such as community dialogues, and are natural places to embed the skills and resources needed for deliberation. To create a culture of deliberative dialogue and decision-making, it needs to become routine practice at key junctures of health sector decision-making. Having a network of organizations with deliberative expertise could also be operationalized when faced with the next pandemic, which surely is in our future.

CONCLUSION

The nation's declining health and its health inequalities concern health experts. We believe meaningful and informed deliberation among citizens to learn and problem solve together is one promising remedy to our nation's ills. Public deliberation is not cheap, but the costs of a sick and polarized nation are far greater. A serious investment in the nation's civic health just might improve the nation's population health. AJPH

CORRESPONDENCE

Correspondence should be sent to Erika Blacksher, 1111 Main St, Suite 500, Kansas City, MO 64105 (e-mail: eblacksher@practicalbioethics.org). Reprints can be ordered at http://www.ajph.org by clicking the "Reprints" link.

PUBLICATION INFORMATION

Full Citation: Blacksher E, Asada Y, Danis M, Gold MR, Kassebaum N, Onge JS. Building a "we" with deliberative dialogue in pursuit of health for all. *Am J Public Health*. 2023;113(10):1110–1113.

Acceptance Date: July 11, 2023.

DOI: https://doi.org/10.2105/AJPH.2023.307392

CONTRIBUTORS

E. Blacksher wrote the original manuscript, incorporated reviews, and finalized the manuscript. All authors contributed to the conceptualization of the article, provided substantive reviews, and approved the final version.

ACKNOWLEGEMENTS

The project was supported by a grant from the County Health Rankings and Roadmaps program, a program of the University of Wisconsin Population Health Institute with support from the Robert Wood Johnson Foundation (grant 78090). The project was also supported in part by the Intramural Research Program of the National Institutes of Health.

Y. Asada, E. Blacksher, M. Danis, and M. R. Gold collectively have 65 years of experience in the design and implementation of democratic deliberation on questions of health and health care. Special thanks go to expert advisors to the project that inspired this article.

Note. The views expressed are those of the authors and do not necessarily reflect the views of the County Health Rankings and Roadmaps program, the Robert Wood Johnson Foundation, the National Institutes of Health, the Department of Health and Human Services, or the US government.

CONFLICTS OF INTEREST

The authors have no conflicts of interest to disclose.

REFERENCES

1. National Research Council and Institute of Medicine. *US Health in International Perspective: Shorter Lives, Poorer Health*. Washington, DC: National Academies Press; 2013.
2. Beckfield J, Bambra C. Shorter lives in stingier states: social policy shortcomings help explain the US mortality disadvantage. *Soc Sci Med*. 2016;171:30–38. https://doi.org/10.1016/j.socscimed.2016.10.017
3. Montez JK, Beckfield J, Cooney JK, et al. US state policies, politics, and life expectancy. *Milbank Q*. 2020;98(3):668–699. https://doi.org/10.1111/1468-0009.12469
4. Montez JK, Mehri N, Monnat SM, et al. US state policy contexts and mortality of working-age adults. *PLoS One*. 2022;17(10):e0275466. https://doi.org/10.1371/journal.pone.0275466
5. Woolf SH. The growing influence of state governments on population health in the United States. *JAMA*. 2022;327(14):1331–1332. https://doi.org/10.1001/jama.2022.3785
6. Burkhalter S, Gastil J, Kelshaw T. A conceptual definition and theoretical model of public deliberation in small face-to-face groups. *Commun Theory*. 2002;12(4):398–422. https://doi.org/10.1111/j.1468-2885.2002.tb00276.x
7. Carpini M, Cook F, Jacobs L. Public deliberation, discursive participation, and citizen engagement: a review of the empirical literature. *Annu Rev Polit Sci*. 2004;7(1):315–344. https://doi.org/10.1146/annurev.polisci.7.121003.091630
8. Goold SD, Biddle AK, Klipp G, Hall CN, Danis M. Choosing Healthplans All Together: a deliberative exercise for allocating limited health care resources. *J Health Polit Policy Law*. 2005;30(4):563–601. https://doi.org/10.1215/03616878-30-4-563
9. Gastil J, Bacci C, Dollinger M. Is deliberation neutral? Patterns of attitude change during "The Deliberative Polls™." *J Deliberative Democracy*. 2010;6(2). https://doi.org/10.16997/jdd.107
10. Luskin RC, O'Flynn I, Fishkin JS, Russell D. Deliberating across deep divides. *Polit Stud*. 2014;62(1):116–135. https://doi.org/10.1111/j.1467-9248.2012.01005.x
11. Fishkin J, Siu A, Diamond L, Bradburn N. Is deliberation an antidote to extreme partisan polarization? Reflections on "America in One Room." *Am Polit Sci Rev*. 2021;115(4):1464–1481. https://doi.org/10.1017/S0003055421000642
12. Ugarriza JE, Nussio E. There is no pill for deliberation: explaining discourse quality in post-conflict communities. *Schweiz Z Polit*. 2016;22(1):145–166. https://doi.org/10.1111/spsr.12195
13. Carman K, Maurer M, Mallery C, et al. *Community Forum Deliberative Methods Demonstration: Evaluating Effectiveness and Eliciting Public Views on Use*

of Evidence. Rockville, MD: Agency for Healthcare Research and Quality; 2014. AHRQ publication no. 14(15)-EHC007-EF. https://doi.org/10.2139/ssrn.3123559.

14. Wang G, Gold M, Siegel J, et al. Deliberation: obtaining informed input from a diverse public. *J Health Care Poor Underserved*. 2015;26(1):223–242. https://doi.org/10.1353/hpu.2015.0021
15. Blacksher E, Diebel A, Forest PG, Goold SD, Abelson J. What is public deliberation? *Hastings Cent Rep*. 2012;42(2):14–17. https://doi.org/10.1002/hast.26
16. Abelson J, Blacksher EA, Li KK, Boesveld SE, Goold SD. Public deliberation in health policy and bioethics: mapping an emerging, interdisciplinary field. *J Deliberative Democracy*. 2013;9(1). https://doi.org/10.16997/jdd.157
17. Davies C, Barnett E, Wetherell M, Seymour-Smith S. *Opening the Box: Evaluating the Citizens Council of NICE*. Milton Keynes, UK: The Open University; 2005.
18. Scherer M, Kamler A, Weiss L, Blacksher E, Jeavons J, Gold MR. Using public deliberation to set priorities: the case of COVID-19 vaccine access in New York City. *J Public Health Manag Pract*. 2022;28(1):86–94. https://doi.org/10.1097/PHH.0000000000001471
19. Danis M, Kotwani N, Garrett J, Rivera I, Davies-Cole J, Carter-Nolan P. Priorities of low-income urban residents for interventions to address the socio-economic determinants of health. *J Health Care Poor Underserved*. 2010;21(4):1318–1339. https://doi.org/10.1353/hpu.2010.0929
20. Subica AM, Brown BJ. Addressing health disparities through deliberative methods: citizens' panels for health equity. *Am J Public Health*. 2020;110(2):166–173. https://doi.org/10.2105/AJPH.2019.305450
21. Kamler A, Weiss L, Chittum C, Owusu S, Gold MR. Public deliberation in service to health equity: investing resources in Roanoke, Virginia. *NAM Perspect*. 2020;2020:10.31478/202008d. https://doi.org/10.31478/202008d
22. Robert SA, Booske BC. US opinions on health determinants and social policy as health policy. *Am J Public Health*. 2011;101(9):1655–1663. https://doi.org/10.2105/AJPH.2011.300217
23. Carger E, Westen D, Robert Wood Johnson Foundation. A new way to talk about the social determinants of health. 2010. Available at: https://www.rwjf.org/en/library/research/2010/01/a-new-way-to-talk-about-the-social-determinants-of-health.html. Accessed January 6, 2022.
24. Gollust SE, Lantz PM, Ubel PA. The polarizing effect of news media messages about the social determinants of health. *Am J Public Health*. 2009;99(12):2160–2167. https://doi.org/10.2105/AJPH.2009.161414
25. Lundell H, Niederdeppe J, Clarke C. Public views about health causation, attributions of responsibility, and inequality. *J Health Commun*. 2013;18(9):1116–1130. https://doi.org/10.1080/10810730.2013.768724
26. Gollust SE, Lynch J. Who deserves health care? The effects of causal attributions and group cues on public attitudes about responsibility for health care costs. *J Health Polit Policy Law*. 2011;36(6):1061–1095. https://doi.org/10.1215/03616878-1460578
27. Niederdeppe J, Bu QL, Borah P, Kindig DA, Robert SA. Message design strategies to raise public awareness of social determinants of health and population health disparities. *Milbank Q*. 2008;86(3):481–513. https://doi.org/10.1111/j.1468-0009.2008.00530.x
28. Cooper LA, Roter DL, Johnson RL, Ford DE, Steinwachs DM, Powe NR. Patient-centered communication, ratings of care, and concordance of patient and physician race. *Ann Intern Med*. 2003;139(11):907–915. https://doi.org/10.7326/0003-4819-139-11-200312020-00009

Generation Z Challenges Partisan Divides for Health Equity

Philip M. Alberti, PhD, Kendal Orgera, MPH, MPP, and Carla S. Alvarado, PhD, MPH

ABOUT THE AUTHORS

Philip M. Alberti is senior director, Health Equity Research and Policy, Association of American Medical Colleges (AAMC), Washington, DC. Philip M. Alberti is also founding director, and Carla S. Alvarado is director of research, Center for Health Justice, AAMC. Kendal Orgera is senior research analyst, Research and Action Institute, AAMC.

See also Building Common Ground, pp. 1093–1115.

AJPH October 2023, Vol 113, No. 10

By its very definition, "health equity"—a state where every community has an equal opportunity to thrive—is for everyone. No community should face unjust and avoidable barriers to the basic, vital conditions[1] (humane housing, reliable transportation, quality health care, etc.) we all need to be healthy and well. Nor is health equity a zero-sum game with winners and losers: we all stand to gain. Yet despite the universal benefit, finding common ground for the kinds of laws and policies that would achieve health equity seems impossible given our entrenched political divides. As a result, health equity remains an ideal for some future, better, and healthier United States.

That future will be shaped not only by those of us currently in political power but also by generations to follow, starting with Generation Z (Gen Z). Of late, much has been made about that group's burgeoning political muscle. In recent elections, young voters have "connected the dots between movement insurgency and voter mobilization" in ways that "could be a game changer."[2]

In December 2022, the Association of American Medical Colleges, Center for Health Justice conducted a nationally representative poll of members of Gen Z, aged 18–24 years, to identify emerging areas of multiracial, bipartisan, cross-geography and -demography consensus on topics relevant to achieving health equity.[3] Given current political debates, we were surprised by unexpected areas of agreement among these younger self-identified Democrats, Independents, and Republicans.

Although 10 states have still not expanded Medicaid,[4] 76% of Republican Gen Zers agreed with Democrats (93%) and Independents (86%) that access to health care is a basic human right, with more than two thirds of Republicans (68%) saying it is the responsibility of the federal government to ensure that everyone has health care coverage. Although some in Congress recently proposed a regressive flat sales tax to replace the Internal Revenue Service, we saw bipartisan support among Gen Z members for economic policies that instead "try to reduce the gap in wealth between the richest and poorest Americans" (84% D, 70% I, 57% R) and "give economic support to those with lower incomes" (88% D, 74% I, 56% R).[3]

Even where differences remained, surprising areas of common ground emerged. For example, although a majority of Republican Gen Zers (54%), unlike their Democratic (29%) and Independent (37%) counterparts believe that racial health inequities result from individual choices and not systemic racism, all three groups agreed (83% D, 68% I, 60% R) that COVID-19 "highlighted inequities that were already present in the US health care system."[3] Similarly, although 60% of Republican Gen Zers endorsed the idea that "the role that racism plays in our society is overplayed," a majority (55%) agreed with Democrats (89%) and Independents (75%) that it is important that the federal government address "racial residential segregation and discrimination in housing."[3]

Those of us committed to health equity and population health should take these data as a call to action. While we work to overcome current political division and dysfunction, let us also adopt a future-oriented health equity agenda that prioritizes these agreements of tomorrow. Let us build (on) common ground between our future leaders' camps now so that when Gen Z assumes power the distance is shorter and smoother to travel. Health care policy, economic policy, and housing policy may be fertile ground and less about building consensus than about growing and solidifying it.

Specifically, efforts to promote Gen Z agreement on health equity–promoting policy and advocacy should focus on three areas: engagement, state and local action, and creating local to national professional development pathways. First and foremost, there should be intentional, easy ways for youths to be engaged and their voices heard in all aspects of policymaking and movement-building processes. Other recent polling has found that Gen Z is the generation least likely to be proud to live in the United States or to trust its institutions.[5,6] Those of us in power now must demonstrate that we—and the sectors we represent—are worthy of Gen Z's trust and therefore their active participation in the health promotion process. Luckily, models and frameworks exist to create meaningful, trustworthy partnerships and coalitions.[7,8]

Second, given the seemingly intransigent partisanship at the national level, bipartisan health equity movement building must start at the state and local levels and prioritize action where agreement can be most readily mobilized. For example, in our poll, Gen Z strongly agreed across party lines that the government should address the shortage of homes and apartments for rent (89% D, 78% I, 73% R). Housing reform advocates in states as politically disparate as Washington and Montana have had bipartisan success by grounding their work in local perspectives and cultures; for example, the so-called Montana Miracle was achieved by advocating free market reforms that incentivize building affordable housing, such as duplexes, as a way "to conserve rural areas and avoid Los Angeles–style sprawl."[9] A locally resonant message developed through authentic engagement can catalyze action on topics important to Gen Z across party lines, easing the path to their participation and power.

Finally, to develop local leaders into national ones and ensure that scarce resources are equitably deployed, we must intentionally connect local, state, and national action and create professional development opportunities that span the three. For example, our poll found bipartisan agreement among Gen Zers that climate change was both an immediate (84% D, 71% I, 56% R) and long-term (90% D, 75% I, 64% R) threat to the safety of the planet. As of 2021, 11 mostly "blue" states had passed environmental justice legislation and an additional 11 mostly "red" and "purple" states had such legislation pending.[10] Strengthening formal connections among national youth-led environmental organizations like the Sunrise Movement, and these state environmental justice efforts can maximize resources, help with the bidirectional amplification and spreading of successes, and create a pathway for the next generation of national health equity leaders.

By some measures, the United States is the wealthiest nation in the history of our planet, so health inequities are not inevitable. Our people and government make choices that perpetuate the racial, social, and economic injustices that create them. If we take our cues from Gen Z and focus our efforts on their common ground, perhaps the rising generation will make better, healthier choices for all our communities. AJPH

CORRESPONDENCE

Correspondence should be sent to Philip M. Alberti, PhD, 655 K St NW, Washington, DC 20001 (e-mail: palberti@aamc.org). Reprints can be ordered at: http://www.ajph.org by clicking the "Reprints" link.

PUBLICATION INFORMATION

Full Citation: Alberti PM, Orgera K, Alvarado CS. Generation Z challenges partisan divides for health equity. *Am J Public Health*. 2023;113(10):1114–1115.

Acceptance Date: July 11, 2023.

DOI: https://doi.org/10.2105/AJPH.2023.307391

CONTRIBUTORS

P. M. Alberti created the initial draft of the editorial. K. Orgera conducted the statistical analysis. K. Orgera and C. S. Alvarado developed the polling instrument. All authors interpreted the data and revised the editorial.

CONFLICTS OF INTEREST

The authors have no conflicts of interest to report.

REFERENCES

1. Milstein B, Payne B, Kelleher C, et al. Organizing around vital conditions moves the social determinants agenda into wider action. February 2, 2023. Available at: https://doi.org/10.1377/forefront.20230131.673841. Accessed July 16, 2023.
2. Gash A, Tichenor DJ. Gen Z might finally turn young voters into a political power. *Washington Post*. December 9, 2022. Available at: https://www.washingtonpost.com/made-by-history/2022/12/09/gen-z-activism-voting. Accessed July 16, 2023.
3. Megibow E, Orgera K, Piepenbrink S. Generation Z takes the reins. May 1, 2023. Available at: https://www.aamchealthjustice.org/news/polling/generation-z-takes-reins. Accessed July 16, 2023.
4. Kaiser Family Foundation. Status of state Medicaid expansion decisions: interactive map. December 1, 2022. Available at: https://www.kff.org/medicaid/issue-brief/status-of-state-medicaid-expansion-decisions-interactive-map. Accessed July 7, 2023.
5. Alberti PM, Piepenbrink S. The state of trustworthiness. December 16, 2021. Available at: https://www.aamchealthjustice.org/news/polling/state-trust. Accessed July 7, 2023.
6. Statista. US adults' pride in being American, 2022, by generation. January 23, 2023. Available at: https://www.statista.com/statistics/1359532/share-adults-proud-american-generation-us. Accessed July 5, 2023.
7. Aguilar-Gaxiola S, Ahmed SM, Anise A, et al. Organizing Committee for Assessing Meaningful Community Engagement in Health & Health Care Programs & Policies. Assessing meaningful community engagement: a conceptual model to advance health equity through transformed systems for health. *NAM Perspect*. 2022;2022:10.31478/202202c. [Published online February 14, 2022]. https://doi.org/10.31478/202202c
8. Association of American Medical Colleges, Center for Health Justice. The principles of trustworthiness. Available at: https://www.aamchealthjustice.org/our-work/trustworthiness/trustworthiness-toolkit. Accessed July 5, 2023.
9. Hamilton E. Bipartisan hope for affordable housing emerges in the West. June 20, 2023. Available at: https://www.governing.com/housing/bipartisan-hope-for-affordable-housing-emerges-in-the-west. Accessed July 7, 2023.
10. Bruce D. Analysis: state laws are codifying environmental justice. March 9, 2021. Available at: https://news.bloomberglaw.com/bloomberg-law-analysis/analysis-state-laws-are-codifying-environmental-justice. Accessed July 7, 2023.

Geographic and Sociodemographic Variations in Prevalence of Mental Health Symptoms Among US Youths, 2022

Junxiu Liu, PhD, Zhiyang Zhou, PhD, Xi Cheng, MPH, and Nita Vangeepuram, MD, MPH

AJPH October 2023, Vol 113, No. 10

Objectives. To assess geographic and sociodemographic variations in prevalence of mental health symptoms among US youths.

Methods. We analyzed data from the Household Pulse Survey, phases 3.5 and 3.6, between June 1 and November 14, 2022. The sample included 103 296 households with an estimated 190 017 youths younger than 18 years. We defined mental health symptoms based on parental responses and estimated prevalence by state and subgroups, including race/ethnicity, parental education, household income, housing tenure, household food sufficiency, and health insurance coverage. All analyses incorporated sampling weight.

Results. An estimated 34.5% (95% confidence interval [CI] = 33.7%, 35.3%) of youths had parent-reported mental health symptoms. The prevalence of symptoms varied across states, ranging from 27.9% (95% CI = 23.8%, 32.0%) in Florida to 46.4% (95% CI = 41.9%, 50.9%) in New Hampshire. We observed variations by subgroup, with youths in households that did not pay rent reporting a prevalence of 43.8% (95% CI = 39.3%, 48.4%) and those experiencing food insufficiency reporting a prevalence of 56.0% (95% CI = 50.9%, 61.2%).

Conclusions. There is an urgent need for attention to mental health challenges among youths, taking into account geographic and sociodemographic variations. (*Am J Public Health*. 2023;113(10):1116–1119. https://doi.org/10.2105/AJPH.2023.307355)

There has been a growing concern regarding youths' mental health, with an increasing prevalence of symptoms over the past decade and further exacerbation during the COVID-19 pandemic.[1–3] According to a US Centers for Disease Control and Prevention report, more than a third of high school students reported mental health challenges during the pandemic.[4] In a 2022 Pew Research Center survey, 40% of US parents listed mental health as a top concern for their children.[5] In October 2022, the US Preventive Services Task Force released a recommendation for anxiety screening in children and adolescents aged 8 to 18 years based on the comprehensive evaluation of existing evidence and the need for timely detection and intervention.[6] Because of the rising trend in prevalence of mental health symptoms, widespread concerns have been observed globally.[3] However, the current knowledge regarding geographic and sociodemographic variations in the prevalence of these symptoms among US youths remains limited.

We examined geographic and sociodemographic variations in the prevalence of mental health symptoms among US youths younger than 18 years in 2022.

METHODS

The Household Pulse Survey (HPS) is a nationally representative survey conducted by the US Census Bureau in collaboration with multiple federal agencies to collect data on the social and economic effects of the COVID-19 pandemic on US households and to measure household experiences during the pandemic and recovery. We included phases 3.5 and 3.6 (earlier phases of HPS did not have information on youths' mental health), which were conducted between June 1 and November 14, 2022. Among 322 361 households, we included 103 296 households with an estimated population of 190 017 youths younger than 18 years. We defined the presence of mental health symptoms among youths as positive responses by parents or caregivers to either of the questions "In the past 4 weeks, did any children living in your household: 1) 'feel anxious or clingy' or 2) 'feel very sad or depressed?'"

Although the data collected by the HPS was at the household level, we followed the technical documentation of the HPS to generate individual-level estimates for youths.[7] Specifically, we adjusted the final HPS person weights offered by the US Census Bureau by multiplying them by the ratio of the number of adults to the number of children that were reported to live in each household (see Appendix [available as a supplement to the online version of this article at http://www.ajph.org]). As a result, the constructed weights accounted for household nonresponse, the number of children per household, and the sampling coverage.

Using these weights, we estimated the outcomes of interest via a Hájek-type estimator accounting for nonresponses to the questions regarding youths' mental health symptoms.[8] We constructed 95% confidence intervals (CIs) following Fay's method of balanced repeated replication, as suggested by the Census Bureau.[9] For subgroup analyses, we included race/ethnicity (Hispanic, non-Hispanic Asian, non-Hispanic Black, non-Hispanic White, and other), parental educational level, household income level, housing tenure, household food sufficiency, health insurance coverage, and geographic region.

RESULTS

In 2022, an estimated 34.5% (95% CI = 33.7%, 35.3%) of youths reported experiencing mental health symptoms. The prevalence of symptoms varied significantly across states, ranging from 27.9% (95% CI = 23.8%, 32.0%) in Florida to 46.4% (95% CI = 41.9%, 50.9%) in New Hampshire (Appendix Table A and Figure A). Moreover, there were significant variations in the prevalence of mental health symptoms observed in sociodemographic subgroups (Table 1). For example, the prevalence of symptoms was 22.6% (95% CI = 19.9%, 27.3%) among non-Hispanic Asian youths, 28.5% (95% CI = 26.2%, 30.7%) among non-Hispanic Black youths, 32.2% (95% CI = 29.6%, 34.8%) among Hispanic youths, 37.7% (95% CI = 36.8%, 38.5%) among non-Hispanic White youths, and 41.0% (95% CI = 37.6%, 44.4%) among others.

Youths with parents with higher education had more mental health symptoms; the prevalence of mental health symptom was 37.4% (95% CI = 36.3%, 38.5%) among youths whose parents had graduate degrees compared with 30.3% (95% CI = 23.8%, 36.8%) among those whose parents had less than a high school–level education. By contrast, youths from households with the highest income level (≥ $200 000) had a lower prevalence of mental health symptoms at 30.7% (95% CI = 29.1%, 32.3%) than did those from households with the lowest income level (< $25 000) at 37.3% (95% CI = 34.8%, 39.8%). The prevalence of mental health symptoms varied by housing status, with a lower prevalence of 29.5% (95% CI = 27.2%, 31.7%) observed among youths from households who owned their housing free and clear and with a higher prevalence of 49.0% (95% CI = 40.8%, 57.3%) observed among youths from household units occupied without rent payments.

Furthermore, the prevalence of mental health symptoms was 58.0% (95% CI = 51.7%, 64.2%) among youths who frequently experienced food insufficiency, which was more than double the prevalence observed among those who did not: 26.3% (95% CI = 25.4%, 27.1%). Prevalence of mental health symptoms also differed by household health insurance coverage, with a higher prevalence of 37.7% (95% CI = 36.1%, 39.2%) observed among youths with public health insurance compared with a prevalence of 34.4% (95% CI = 32.6%, 34.3%) among youths with private health insurance. We also estimated the number of youths affected by mental health symptoms by state (Appendix Table A) and sociodemographic subgroup (Table 1).

DISCUSSION

We found that more than a third of US youths experienced mental health symptoms in 2022, with substantial variations observed across states (from 27.9% in Florida to 46.4% in New Hampshire) and sociodemographic subgroups (from 26.3% for youths who had enough and satisfactory food to 58.0% for those who frequently experienced insufficient food). Research on mental health among children and adolescents during the pandemic is sparse, and comparability of estimates across studies is challenging because of

TABLE 1— Prevalence of Mental Health Symptoms and Number of Affected Individuals by Sociodemographic Factors Among US Youths Aged < 18 Years: Household Pulse Survey, 2022

Characteristic	Prevalence Estimate, % (95% CI)	No., Millions, Estimate (95% CI)
Race/ethnicity		
Hispanic	32.2 (29.6, 34.8)	5.4 (4.9, 5.8)
Non-Hispanic Asian	22.6 (19.9, 27.3)	0.9 (0.7, 1.1)
Non-Hispanic Black	28.5 (26.2, 30.7)	3.3 (3.0, 3.6)
Non-Hispanic White	37.7 (36.8, 38.5)	15.2 (14.8, 15.5)
Other	41.0 (37.6, 44.4)	1.5 (1.4, 1.6)
Parental education		
< high school	30.3 (23.8, 36.8)	0.9 (0.7, 1.1)
Some high school	28.8 (23.5, 34.1)	1.5 (1.2, 1.8)
High school graduate or equivalent	29.3 (27.5, 31.2)	7.0 (6.6, 7.4)
Some college	38.0 (36.2, 39.8)	5.8 (5.6, 6.1)
Associate's degree	39.3 (37.4, 41.3)	2.7 (2.6, 2.9)
Bachelor's degree	37.3 (36.1, 38.4)	4.3 (4.2, 4.5)
Graduate degree	37.4 (36.3, 38.5)	3.9 (3.8, 4.1)
Household income level, $		
< 25 000	37.3 (34.8, 39.8)	4.1 (3.7, 4.4)
25 000–34 999	36.3 (33.1, 39.4)	3.0 (2.7, 3.3)
35 000–49 999	35.2 (32.7, 37.7)	3.0 (2.8, 3.2)
50 000–74 999	34.3 (31.9, 36.7)	3.8 (3.6, 4.1)
75 000–99 999	34.4 (32.3, 36.5)	2.8 (2.7, 3.0)
100 000–149 999	35.1 (33.3, 36.9)	3.6 (3.4, 3.8)
150 000–199 999	34.2 (31.9, 36.5)	1.8 (1.6, 1.9)
≥ 200 000	30.7 (29.1, 32.3)	2.1 (2.0, 2.2)
Housing tenure		
Owned by you or someone in this household free and clear	29.5 (27.2, 31.7)	3.1 (2.9, 3.4)
Owned by you or someone in the household with a mortgage or loan, including home equity loans	34.8 (33.9, 35.7)	13.1 (12.7, 13.5)
Rented	35.2 (33.5, 37.0)	8.5 (8.0, 9.0)
Occupied without payment of rent	49.0 (40.8, 57.3)	0.7 (0.5, 0.9)
Household food sufficiency for last 7 d		
Enough	26.3 (25.4, 27.1)	9.9 (9.5, 10.2)
Enough, but not always	38.9 (37.3, 40.5)	10.4 (9.9, 10.9)
Sometimes not enough	46.3 (43.2, 49.3)	4.3 (4.0, 4.6)
Often not enough	58.0 (51.7, 64.2)	1.6 (1.4, 1.9)
Public insurance coverage		
Yes	37.7 (36.1, 39.2)	9.7 (9.2, 10.2)
No	32.9 (32.9, 33.9)	14.9 (14.4, 15.4)
Private insurance coverage		
Yes	34.4 (32.6, 34.3)	17.8 (17.3, 18.2)
No	37.1 (35.4, 38.9)	7.9 (7.4, 8.3)

Note. CI = confidence interval. All estimates and their corresponding 95% CIs are weighted, accounting for the sampling survey design.

differences in age ranges and definitions of mental health symptoms.[10] In addition to national estimates before the pandemic,[11] a recent study[12] found that mental health visits doubled from 2011 to 2020, highlighting the urgent need to prioritize mental health among the youth population. Our study further provides new insight into the disparities in mental health across states and sociodemographic characteristics.

Several limitations in this study need to be noted. First, the assessment of mental health symptoms relied on parental report of symptoms of anxiety and depression over the past 4 weeks, which is not a diagnostic method and may not capture long-term symptoms or other mental health conditions. In addition, because of the lack of individual-level data for youths, we estimated the prevalence of mental health symptoms among youths using personal weights adjustment according to the analytical guideline provided by the US Census Bureau. Despite these limitations, our findings underscore the urgent need to address mental health challenges facing youths in the United States.

Our results highlight the necessity of developing and implementing tailored and targeted interventional programs that take into account geographic and sociodemographic variations in mental health symptoms. Policymakers and health care providers should pay special attention to the subgroups of youths who are disproportionately affected by mental health symptoms, such as those living in households that do not pay rent and those experiencing food insufficiency, and incorporate increased access to youths' mental health resources as part of overall strategies to address broader social determinants of health. AJPH

ABOUT THE AUTHORS

Junxiu Liu and Nita Vangeepuram are with the Department of Population Health Science and Policy, Icahn School of Medicine at Mount Sinai, New York, NY. Zhiyang Zhou is with the Department of Statistics, University of Manitoba, Canada. Xi Cheng is with the Interdisciplinary Program of Science in Analytics, Georgia Institute of Technology, Atlanta. Nita Vangeepuram is also with the Department of Pediatrics, Icahn School of Medicine at Mount Sinai.

CORRESPONDENCE

Correspondence should be sent to Junxiu Liu, PhD, Department of Population Health Science and Policy, Icahn School of Medicine at Mount Sinai, One Gustave L. Levy Place, New York, NY 10029 (e-mail: junxiu.liu@mountsinai.org). Reprints can be ordered at http://www.ajph.org by clicking the "Reprints" link.

PUBLICATION INFORMATION

Full Citation: Liu J, Zhou Z, Cheng X, Vangeepuram N. Geographic and sociodemographic variations in prevalence of mental health symptoms among US youths, 2022. *Am J Public Health*. 2023;113(10):1116–1119.

Acceptance Date: May 23, 2023.

DOI: https://doi.org/10.2105/AJPH.2023.307355

CONTRIBUTORS

J. Liu conceptualized the study, supervised the statistical analyses, and wrote the first draft of the article. J. Liu and N. Vangeepuram critically revised the article. Z. Zhou conducted the statistical analyses and contributed to the writing of the article. X. Cheng prepared the data and figures and conducted the statistical analyses. Z. Zhou and X. Cheng revised the article.

ACKNOWLEDGMENTS

Z. Zhou is financially supported by the Natural Sciences and Engineering Research Council of Canada.

We thank the reviewers and the editorial office for their valuable comments and feedback.

CONFLICTS OF INTEREST

The authors have no conflicts of interest to disclose.

HUMAN PARTICIPANT PROTECTION

Because the data are publicly available and de-identified, institutional review board approval was not required.

REFERENCES

1. Centers for Disease Control and Prevention. Symptoms of anxiety or depressive disorder and use of mental health care among adults during the COVID-19 pandemic—United States, August 2020–February 2021. *MMWR Morb Mortal Wkly Rep*. 2021;70(13):490–494. https://doi.org/10.15585/mmwr.mm7013e2
2. World Health Organization. COVID-19 pandemic triggers 25% increase in prevalence of anxiety and depression worldwide. Available at: https://www.who.int/news/item/02-03-2022-covid-19-pandemic-triggers-25-increase-in-prevalence-of-anxiety-and-depression-worldwide. Accessed May 6, 2023.
3. Sun Y, Wu Y, Fan S, et al. Comparison of mental health symptoms before and during the COVID-19 pandemic: evidence from a systematic review and meta-analysis of 134 cohorts. *BMJ*. 2023;380:e074224. https://doi.org/10.1136/bmj-2022-074224
4. Centers for Disease Control and Prevention. Mental health, suicidality, and connectedness among high school students during the COVID-19 pandemic—Adolescent Behaviors and Experiences Survey, United States, January–June 2021. *MMWR Suppl*. 2022;71(3):16–21. https://doi.org/10.15585/mmwr.su7103a3
5. Pew Research Center. Parenting in America today. January 24, 2023. Available at: https://www.pewresearch.org/social-trends/2023/01/24/parenting-in-america-today. Accessed May 6, 2023.
6. Viswanathan M, Wallace IF, Cook Middleton J, et al. Screening for anxiety in children and adolescents: evidence report and systematic review for the US Preventive Services Task Force. *JAMA*. 2022;328(14):1445–1455. https://doi.org/10.1001/jama.2022.16303
7. US Census Bureau. Household Pulse Survey technical documentation. Available at: https://www.census.gov/programs-surveys/household-pulse-survey/technical-documentation.html. Accessed October 15, 2022.
8. Wu C, Thompson ME. *Sampling Theory and Practice*. Cham, Switzerland: Springer; 2020. https://doi.org/10.1007/978-3-030-44246-0
9. US Census Bureau. Source of the data and accuracy of the estimates for the Household Pulse Survey–phase 3.6. October 15, 2022. Available at: https://www2.census.gov/programs-surveys/demo/technical-documentation/hhp/Phase3-6_Source_and_Accuracy_Week50.pdf. Accessed July 21, 2023.
10. Rider EA, Ansari E, Varrin PH, Sparrow J. Mental health and wellbeing of children and adolescents during the COVID-19 pandemic. *BMJ*. 2021;374:n1730. https://doi.org/10.1136/bmj.n1730
11. Centers for Disease Control and Prevention. Mental health surveillance among children—United States, 2013–2019. *MMWR Suppl*. 2022;71(2):1–42. https://doi.org/10.15585/mmwr.su7102a1
12. Bommersbach TJ, McKean AJ, Olfson M, Rhee TG. National trends in mental health-related emergency department visits among youth, 2011–2020. *JAMA*. 2023;329(17):1469–1477. https://doi.org/10.1001/jama.2023.4809

Communities at Risk for Mpox and Stigmatizing Policies: A Randomized Survey, Republic of Korea, 2022

Yongjin Choi, PhD, MPP, and Ashley M. Fox, PhD, MA

Objectives. To estimate the impact of communicating to the public that men who have sex with men (MSM) are most at risk for mpox on potential stigmatization and risk perception.

Methods. We conducted a survey experiment randomizing exposure to messages about mpox among a sample of the South Korean public (n = 1500) in July 2022. We randomized respondents to receive an informational message about mpox that was (1) a neutral informational message about mpox that did not highlight its origins or risk groups (control group), (2) a message explaining that the virus originated in Africa, or (3) a message emphasizing that MSM are most at risk.

Results. We found that emphasizing that MSM are most at risk increases support for policies that would restrict lesbian, gay, bisexual, transgender/-sexual, queer or questioning–related events by about 7 percentage points compared with the control condition. However, the message describing African origins did not affect support for restricting travel from Africa. Neither changed risk perceptions or willingness to be vaccinated against mpox.

Conclusions. Messages aimed at educating the public about most at-risk groups may trigger increased stigmatization of those groups in ways that could contribute to unnecessary persecution. (*Am J Public Health*. 2023;113(10):1120–1127. https://doi.org/10.2105/AJPH.2023.307347)

AJPH October 2023, Vol 113, No. 10

The World Health Organization declared mpox, previously known as monkeypox, a public health emergency of international concern on July 23, 2022, after it spread to multiple nonendemic countries.[1,2] Presently, in the parts of the world where mpox is newly spreading, those most at risk for acquiring the disease are gay and bisexual men who have sex with men (MSM).[2] To avoid stigmatization, public health messaging initially took a neutral tone that conveyed that mpox is not a sexually transmitted infection and did not emphasize the specific risk groups.[3] However, this messaging has raised complex questions about communicating risk to the public. Public health officials may wish to emphasize who are the most at-risk groups to avoid unnecessary panic by accurately reporting that the risk to the public is not generalized. Additionally, more targeted messaging that specifies those who are most at risk can ensure that they are getting the prevention messages and services they need.[4] On the other hand, messages that convey groups who are the most at risk can potentially contribute to the stigmatization of affected groups, especially when they are already marginalized populations.

As mpox continues to spread and appears to remain clustered in high-risk groups, how to convey risk to the public and target resources while avoiding stigma continues to be a pressing question for public health actors. Moreover, as novel infectious diseases emerge, naming conventions and risk group reporting continue to be vexing issues for public health actors.

Stigma has been defined as an "attribute that is deeply discrediting."[5(p3)] Stigma is exercised through the cooccurrence of labeling and stereotyping in the context of unequal power relations and can result in separation from society, status loss, and discrimination.[6] Although often treated as an individual attribute, disease stigma stems from the social construction of illness in a given society and how this understanding is linked to stereotyped beliefs about categories of the individuals most affected.[7,8] In its most extreme form, "structural stigma"[6] can move from individual and societal attitudes to being codified into law, including the imposition of punitive policies or sanctions on stigmatized groups.[9]

Stigma has often accompanied infectious diseases. Precisely because they are communicable, infectious diseases can lead to the social scapegoating of groups perceived to be the primary source of illness.[10] Disease names, such as the "Spanish flu" and "gay-related immune deficiency," may reinforce the scapegoating and stigmatization of certain groups by conveying connotations of accusation or xenophobia.[7,11] Scapegoating can contribute to acts of violent aggression against persecuted groups.[12] Stigmatized social difference may be used to legitimize the status of dominant social groups at the top of the social hierarchy.[13] Commentators have attributed the increase in anti-Asian hate crimes in the United States during the COVID-19 pandemic to the hateful populist rhetoric reinforcing its East Asian origins (e.g., calling COVID-19 the "China virus" or "Kung Flu").[14]

Once a particular group is associated with a disease, it can lead to overestimating disease prevalence among those who are at heightened risk and underestimating the prevalence among others. For instance, even in countries where MSM are not the primary risk group for HIV, HIV and AIDS are still largely mistakenly associated with this risk group.[15] Furthermore, stigma can contribute to support for policies that violate the civil liberties of affected groups and can lead to further societal ostracization and persecution. Historically, disease epidemics, such as the 1892 typhus and cholera outbreaks in New York City, provoked nativist sentiments culminating in quarantine measures targeting specific ethnic and religious groups and prompting calls to suspend immigration.[10] Public health has long grappled with how to balance the civil rights of individuals and vulnerable groups with the need for restrictive measures to prevent forward transmission of disease.[16] Thus, associating mpox with the sexual behaviors of marginalized risk groups has the potential to downplay the risk of generalized transmission while also increasing support for restrictive measures that might unnecessarily violate civil liberties.

Likewise, because mpox originated in Africa, news stories of the outbreak featuring stock photos of severe cases in African children have raised concerns about the exoticization of the disease in ways that may contribute to "othering" and may excessively heighten fear.[17] During the 2014 Ebola outbreak in West Africa, national media outlets in the United States conceptualized Ebola as a scary and exotic virus by pairing terms that fostered fear of the virus with words that evoked Africa and using alarming images and fear-inducing headlines.[17] This othering process steered the public discourse of the outbreak in a direction that stigmatized Africans living in the United States and people who travel to African countries.[17]

The discourse also contributed to some states adopting non–evidence-based quarantine measures for returning health workers that hampered the Ebola response.[18] Previous research has found that infectious disease outbreaks tend to raise public anxieties in ways that support more restrictive measures than would ordinarily be tolerated because of heightened fear.[19] Thus, media portrayals of mpox as a "foreign" and "African" disease may produce heightened risk perception in ways that may contribute to discriminatory or overly draconian policies.[20]

As in much of the world, in the Republic of Korea (ROK), potentially stigmatizing media coverage of the mpox outbreak preceded the identification of the first case. The coverage consisted of noting the rise of mpox cases in nonendemic countries, the fact that the disease is endemic to Africa, and the unexplained clustering of cases in gay men. The first case of mpox in ROK was confirmed on June 22, 2022, in a Korean citizen returning from Germany. In response, the Korean government raised its alert level to "caution" and pledged to strengthen monitoring and response systems for the disease.[21]

The identification of the first case also coincided with Gay Pride month and preceded the Seoul Queer Culture Festival, which was scheduled for July 16, 2022.[22] Although official reporting stressed that the disease was not sexually transmitted and could only spread through close skin-to-skin contact,[23] some social media discussions called for the cancellation of the queer festival.[22] Homosexuality remains a contentious issue in Korea. According to a 2020 Pew Center Poll, only 44% of Koreans say that homosexuality should be accepted by society compared with 72% in the United States.[24] Thus, we anticipated that the Korean public might be susceptible to messages that identify marginalized risk groups in their support for restrictive policies, particularly those burdening risk groups.

We sought to estimate the impact of communicating to the public the heightened risk among MSM and the disease's African origins on risk perceptions, vaccine acceptance, and support

AJPH October 2023, Vol 113, No. 10

for potentially stigmatizing policies through a survey experiment randomizing exposure to messages about mpox in ROK. Through a survey experiment with a factorial design, we randomly assigned respondents to 5 total treatment groups: 2 message arms (i.e., MSM and African origins) with and without an image that presents the severity of skin lesions as a symptom of mpox.

METHODS

We ran the experiment on a random sample of ROK adults (n = 1500) between July 4 and July 8, 2022, shortly before the public health emergency of international concern was declared and shortly after the first case of mpox received wide media and public attention in the country. Although there were only a few confirmed cases of mpox, ROK is one of the least ethnically diverse countries[25] and has a culture that is relatively less supportive of same-sex marriages.[26] Therefore, the stigmatizing effect of messaging highlighting the African roots and the relevance of sexual minorities to mpox may be more salient in Korean society.

We randomized respondents to receive information about mpox that was (1) a neutral message providing basic information about mpox (control group), (2) a message indicating that the virus originated in Africa, or (3) a message emphasizing that gay and bisexual men are most at risk for contracting mpox. We provided the control group with a neutral, nonstigmatizing message that described the mpox outbreak and was accompanied by an infographic in Korean. The message and infographic explained mpox transition mechanisms, symptoms, and relevant health recommendations and did not refer to risk groups or disease origins.

Additionally, we exposed half of the respondents to an image demonstrating the severity of lesions caused by mpox. The purpose of showing the image was to assess whether demonstrating mpox's severity heightened risk perception and thereby increased support for excessively restrictive and discriminatory policy options. This created 5 treatment conditions and the control group (Table 1). Appendix A (available as a supplement to the online version of this article at http://www.ajph.org) contains the full conditions.

Data

Trend Research, a Korean survey company, collected the data for this study. Trend Research's online panel includes 650 000 members who have opted to receive e-mail invitations to the online survey. The panel is updated twice a year by inviting about 5000 new members. Respondents were selected randomly and stratified by age, gender, and province (including metropolitan city). There were no missing values in the variables used.

Variables

We examined 8 binary outcomes. First, we used 6 binary policy support variables: screening all passengers for symptoms of mpox, requiring all passengers to wear masks on public transportation, beginning mass vaccine production, encouraging people to avoid close contact and stay 6 feet apart in public spaces, banning flights from African countries, and restricting lesbian, gay, bisexual, transgender/-sexual, queer or questioning (LGBTQ) events, such as queer festivals. We measured these variables by using a select all that apply question with 7 choices, including "nothing at this time." These were investigator-created mitigation strategies and did not necessarily represent any government recommendations at the time. Second, we examined a binary measure of respondents' willingness to be vaccinated against mpox. The last outcome variable was risk perception of mpox. We measured this binary variable with a question asking how concerned respondents were about contracting mpox. Appendix B (available as a supplement to the online version of this article at http://www.ajph.org) contains detailed descriptions of the full question wordings and how we coded these variables.

The key independent variable was a categorical factor representing the treatment conditions. Control variables included ideology (liberal, conservative, or independent), age, gender, educational attainment, marital status, job status, having a religion, and monthly household income. We did not report the parameter estimates for these variables in the main results but added them to Appendix D (available as a supplement to the online version of this article at http://www.ajph.org). We did not ask about mpox knowledge because all participants received a standard set of knowledge.

Statistical Analysis

We used ordinary least square regressions with a 95% confidence interval, including the interaction terms between the 2 types of message arms and the image arm, to identify the average treatment effects of each treatment arm in a factorial design. We used 2-tailed statistical tests and completed analyses using Stata version 17 (StataCorp LP, College Station, TX). We used robust SEs for all

TABLE 1— Willingness to Vaccinate Against Mpox, Anxiety About Mpox, Support for Mpox-Related Policies, and Sociodemographics of Survey Respondents, by Treatment Group: Republic of Korea, July 2022

		Treatment 1, %		Treatment 2, %		
Variable	All (n = 1500), %	Without Image[a] (n = 750)	With Image[b] (n = 750)	Plain Description[c] (n = 500)	African Arm[d] (n = 500)	MSM Arm[e] (n = 500)
Willing to vaccinate	45.07	43.73	46.40	44.20	47.20	43.80
Worry about the mpox infection	9.13	9.20	9.07	10.00	9.40	8.00
Support for						
Korea entry inspection	59.13	57.60	60.67	57.40	61.20	58.80
Masks in public transportation	38.47	36.67	40.27	40.60	37.00	37.80
Social distancing	34.73	33.73	35.73	34.40	31.20	38.60
Vaccine production	24.13	23.60	24.67	24.20	24.40	23.80
Travel ban from Africa	33.20	33.60	32.80	33.20	31.40	35.00
Restrictions on LGBTQ events	38.40	37.33	39.47	34.80	38.20	42.20
Political propensity						
Liberal	24.87	23.07	26.67	23.20	26.00	25.40
Independent	22.13	24.00	20.27	23.40	19.80	23.20
Conservative	53.00	52.93	53.07	53.40	54.20	51.40
Woman	49.00	48.40	49.60	45.60	51.80	49.60
Age, y						
18–29	19.53	20.27	18.80	19.20	20.00	19.40
30–39	17.53	17.20	17.87	18.40	17.60	16.60
40–49	21.27	21.87	20.67	20.00	21.00	22.80
50–59	22.60	22.27	22.93	22.60	23.00	22.20
60–69	19.07	18.40	19.73	19.80	18.40	19.00
Education						
High school or less	20.80	18.67	22.93	18.40	19.80	24.20
Bachelor's degree	65.33	68.53	62.13	68.20	66.00	61.80
Master's degree or more	13.87	12.80	14.93	13.40	14.20	14.00
Religiosity	46.00	46.27	45.73	46.40	44.80	46.80
Married	54.60	54.27	54.93	56.40	53.40	54.00
Job status						
Health care workers	6.87	7.33	6.40	7.00	7.20	6.40
Employees	53.40	54.67	52.13	51.40	55.00	53.80
Unemployed/other	39.73	38.00	41.47	41.60	37.80	39.80
Monthly income, ₩, millions						
< 2	11.80	9.60	14.00	12.20	11.40	11.80
2–3.99	31.93	32.13	31.73	29.00	35.40	31.40
4–5.99	27.80	27.33	28.27	30.00	24.60	28.80
6–7.99	14.67	16.53	12.80	14.60	14.80	14.60
> 7.99	13.80	14.40	13.20	14.20	13.80	13.40
No. of responses	1500	750	750	500	500	500

Note. LGBTQ = lesbian, gay, bisexual, transgender/-sexual, queer or questioning; MSM = men who have sex with men.

[a]Participants who were not exposed to an image demonstrating the severity of lesions caused by mpox.
[b]Participants who were exposed to an image demonstrating the severity of lesions caused by mpox.
[c]Participants who received a neutral message providing basic information about mpox.
[d]Participants who received a message including a prompt that mpox originated in Africa.
[e]Participants who received a message including a prompt that gay and bisexual men are most at risk for mpox.

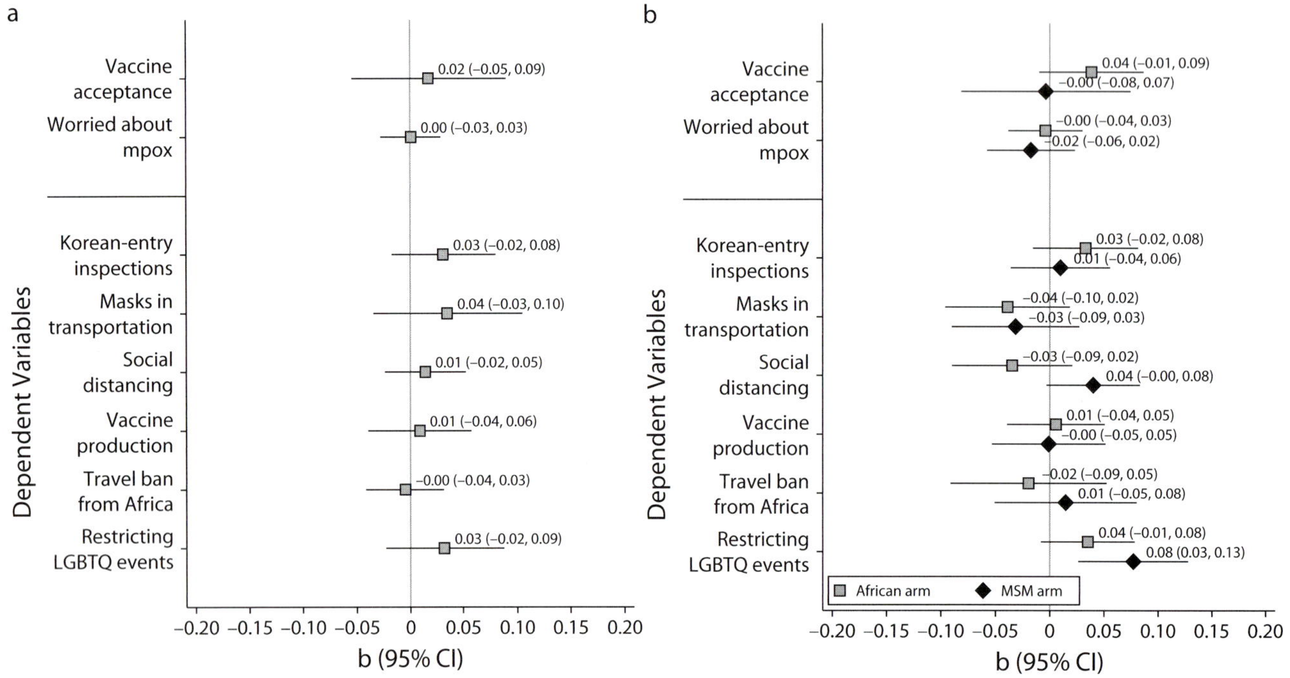

FIGURE 1— Marginal Effects on Stigmatization and Risk Perception of (a) Lesions Image, and (b) Stigmatizing Descriptions: Republic of Korea, July 2022

Note. CI = confidence interval; LGBTQ = lesbian, gay, bisexual, transgender/-sexual, queer or questioning; MSM = men who have sex with men. Results are from an ordinary least squares model. Markers indicate the marginal effect of the experimental arms on the answer. Whiskers and numbers in parentheses indicate 95% CIs. The controls included but not shown are age, gender, educational attainment, marital status, job status, religiosity, and household income.

estimations. Appendix C (available as a supplement to the online version of this article at http://www.ajph.org) provides the full equation with detailed explanations of how we calculated the marginal effects.

RESULTS

Table 1 summarizes the data. Overall, 45% of the sample was willing to be vaccinated against mpox if recommended, and only 9% were worried about getting mpox. Although the majority of the respondents did not support restrictive or stigmatizing policies against mpox, a large portion of respondents did support these policies: 38% supported restricting LGBTQ events and 33% supported banning travel from Africa; 59% also supported entry inspection, 38% masks in public transit, 35% social distancing, and 24% mass mpox vaccine production.

When compared with the 2020 benchmark data from Statistics Korea, our sample showed great consistency with population estimates in terms of gender and age, as we stratified the data collection (Appendix E, available as a supplement to the online version of this article at http://www.ajph.org). The percentage married was slightly lower than the benchmark data but still comparable. However, the study sample tended to oversample more highly educated individuals compared with the benchmark.

Figure 1 presents the average treatment effects of the treatment arms (Appendix D provides the full regression table). We found that exposure to the message emphasizing MSM's risk increased support for restricting LGBTQ-related events by nearly 7 percentage points (35% vs 42%) compared with the control condition. In adjusted ordinary least squares models, this was the only significant result across the study arms and outcomes (8 percentage points; 95% confidence interval [CI] = 0.03, 0.13; $P = .003$; Figure 1b). However, neither the African origin arm nor the MSM arm made a difference in support for banning flights from African countries, willingness to be vaccinated against mpox, anxiety about the mpox infection, or support for other types of policy measures. Exposure to the skin lesions image did not produce any significant differences across the study arms (Figure 1a).

The interaction between the message arms and the image arm was also statistically insignificant (Appendix D). The effect of the MSM arm on the likelihood of support for policies restricting LGBTQ events was stronger when it was presented without the lesions image than with the image (Appendix F, available as a supplement to the online version of this article at http://www.ajph.org). These findings remained the same when estimating based on logistic regression (Appendix G, available as a supplement to the online version of this article at http://www.ajph.org).

The likelihood of endorsing stigmatizing policies was associated with respondents' gender and age (Appendix D). Female respondents were more likely to support banning flights from African countries by 7 percentage points (95% CI = 0.02, 0.11; $P = .006$) than were male respondents.

Compared with politically liberal respondents, politically conservative respondents were more likely to support banning travel from Africa by 7 percentage points (95% CI = 0.01, 0.12; $P = .018$) and restricting LGBTQ events by 12 percentage points (95% CI = 0.02, 0.21; $P = .015$). Politically independent respondents were 8 percentage points more likely to support banning travel from Africa (95% CI = 0.02, 0.13; $P = .007$) and restricting LGBTQ events (95% CI = 0.01, 0.15; $P = .032$) than were liberal respondents. Respondents who are religious were more likely to support banning travel from Africa by 7 percentage points (95% CI = 0.03, 0.11; $P = .001$) and restricting LGBTQ events by 7 percentage points (95% CI = 0.02, 0.11; $P = .010$).

The likelihood of support for banning travel from Africa decreased with respondents' age. Respondents in their 40s (−10 percentage points; 95% CI = −0.17, −0.04; $P = .004$), 50s (−16 percentage points; 95% CI = −0.24, −0.09; $P < .001$), and 60s (−18 percentage points; 95% CI = −0.26, −0.10; $P < .001$) were less supportive of banning travel from Africa than the reference group aged 18 to 29 years. The likelihood of support for restricting LGBTQ events was not significantly associated with age, however.

DISCUSSION

Despite low personal risk perception of mpox in ROK, we found that exposure to a simple prompt emphasizing MSM's risk for mpox increased support for restrictive measures for LGBTQ populations. We found that although only 9% of the sample reported being worried about mpox, individuals who were exposed to a message mentioning MSM's risk for mpox were 8 percentage points more likely to support restricting LGBTQ events when controlling for other covariates. The message did not affect being worried about mpox, vaccine acceptance, or support for other, more generalized mitigation measures, suggesting that adding this information primarily serves to channel stigma rather than to affect risk perception.

Exposure to images showing the severity of lesions did not affect outcomes. The findings are more meaningful because we conducted our study at a time when mpox was not objectively a broad threat to the public, with only 1 identified case in the country at the time of the survey, although the issue was salient in the media. Considering that stigmatizing attitudes can be triggered by a simple vignette in a context in which the public's fear of mpox is moderate, the stigmatizing effects of media messaging might be much greater when the public's risk perception of an infectious disease is more elevated.

We did not find support for the notion that the disease's African origins increased support for policy restrictions that may be associated with xenophobia. Neither the study arm that mentioned the disease's origins in Africa nor the image depicting the severity of lesions increased support for restricting travel from Africa, risk perception, or willingness to be vaccinated, contrary to our hypothesis that images or messages that "exoticized" the illness might unduly affect attitudes. Nevertheless, one third of respondents did support policies to restrict travel from Africa even though travel restrictions contravened the government's messages.[23] These findings are aligned with findings from a study in the United States fielded during the Ebola crisis, which indicated that a simple mention identifying African travelers as the disease carrier in the United States did not make a significant difference in policy preferences.[27]

We did find support for the idea that a simple prompt merely identifying MSM as those most at risk increased support for restricting LGBTQ festivals (an 8 percentage point increase in the likelihood). Although the majority of the public did not endorse these restrictions (62% in the sample), the finding suggests that caution in messaging is needed to carefully take the social ramifications of highlighting risk groups into account in public vaccine communication. Given that the MSM community perceived media reports on mpox to be stigmatizing,[28] crafting more sensitive messages can also help reduce self-stigma in the community.

Those most supportive of restricting LGBTQ events and limiting travel from Africa included older respondents, especially those aged 50 years or older, and women. The higher support among the older generation presumably reflects their lower overall acceptance of homosexuality.[29] However, it is less clear why female respondents in this study were more inclined to favor regulating LGBTQ-related events. Women were also more likely to support more draconian measures, including social distancing and banning flights from Africa, but less likely to support more routine surveillance measures, such as airport screening (Appendix D). This suggests that women in the Korean context may have a greater tendency to place public safety above individual rights. Consistent with this finding, previous studies have found heightened vaccine hesitancy among women in Korea[30] but a greater likelihood of engaging in other preventive behaviors.[31]

Overall, respondents were quite supportive of a variety of mitigation measures despite their low risk perception, with 45% reporting they would be willing to be vaccinated against the disease. Presently, generalized vaccination is not recommended, and vaccination efforts in the United States are limited to the populations most at risk.[32] Large portions of the public also supported entry inspection (nearly 60%), masks in public transit (nearly 40%), social distancing (nearly 35%), and increased vaccine production to prevent the spread of mpox should it become necessary (nearly 25%), although these measures are not currently and never were broadly recommended.

Although we found that emphasizing certain risk groups increased support for potentially discriminatory policies, this does not necessarily suggest that emphasizing generalized risk is a good alternative. Emphasizing generalized risk can cause unnecessary fear and panic that could contribute to further stigmatization of "index" groups—those perceived as having initially introduced a disease—or those who may serve as "bridge" populations to the general public.[33] Current research suggests that the epidemiology of mpox has changed, so that the generalized risk is reduced, and that focusing on the most at-risk groups may be warranted.[34] Thinking beyond mpox, public health practitioners should continue to think carefully about how to present disease origins, disease naming conventions, and whether and when to publicly identify particular risk groups. The extent of marginalization of the primary risk group should be an active consideration. The renaming of monkeypox as mpox is an example of a deliberate strategy to reduce undue fear and anticipate public anxiety.[35] However, decisions need to be proactive rather than reactive.

Limitations

Our study had certain limitations that must be acknowledged. Results in the Korean context might not be broadly generalizable to other contexts. The images used in the image arms were selected to represent what mpox might look like on Asian skin tones and represented relatively mild lesions. The use of more "shocking" stock photos depicting a severe case on African skin tones might have produced a more substantial reaction from the public than what we detected. That 38% of the sample reported supporting restrictions on LGBTQ events suggests there may be high existing stigma toward MSM in ROK, potentially affecting the magnitude of the study results. When the survey was administered, ROK had experienced only 1 domestic case of mpox.

Furthermore, we used only 1 item to assess measures related to treatment of the MSM community. However, the results also speak more broadly to public tolerance of restrictive measures and risk perceptions as they pertain to mpox. Lastly, even though we stratified the sampling, the survey undersampled less educated people and the data might not be free from selection bias because the online panel was more accessible to people with Internet access.

Conclusions

We found that concerns that highlighting MSM's risk might increase stigma are not unfounded. The need to alert the most at-risk groups should be balanced with the possibility of heightened stigma. How to most accurately and appropriately present health threats to the public to raise appropriate risk perceptions and compliance remains an ongoing global challenge for public health. AJPH

ABOUT THE AUTHORS

Yongjin Choi is with the Department of Infectious Disease Epidemiology, London School of Hygiene and Tropical Medicine, London, UK. Ashley M. Fox is with the Department of Public Administration and Policy, University at Albany, State University of New York, Albany.

CORRESPONDENCE

Correspondence should be sent to Yongjin Choi, Department of Infectious Disease Epidemiology, London School of Hygiene and Tropical Medicine, Keppel St, London WC1E 7HT, United Kingdom (e-mail: yongjin.choi@lshtm.ac.uk). Reprints can be ordered at http://www.ajph.org by clicking the "Reprints" link.

PUBLICATION INFORMATION

Full Citation: Choi Y, Fox AM. Communities at risk for mpox and stigmatizing policies: a randomized survey, Republic of Korea, 2022. *Am J Public Health*. 2023;113(10):1120–1127.

Acceptance Date: May 18, 2023.

DOI: https://doi.org/10.2105/AJPH.2023.307347

CONTRIBUTORS

Y. Choi conducted the data analysis. Both authors conceptualized the study, designed the data collection, secured funding, accessed the data, contributed to writing the article, and interpreted the results.

ACKNOWLEDGMENTS

The authors gratefully acknowledge support from the Korean Studies Grant 2022 of the Academy of Korean Studies (grant AKS-2022-R124).

We also thank collaborators on this project: Soohyun Park at University at Albany, State University of New York; Youngsung Kim at Colorado University; Byoung Joon Kim at Kookmin University; and Jinwoo Lee at the Korean Educational Development Institute.

Note. The funder had no role in study design, data collection, analysis, writing, or interpretation of the findings.

CONFLICTS OF INTEREST

The authors have no conflicts of interest to declare.

HUMAN PARTICIPANT PROTECTION

The data collection of this study was reviewed and approved by the institutional review board of the University at Albany, State University of New York (protocol number 22X058).

REFERENCES

1. Del Rio C, Malani PN. Update on the monkeypox outbreak. *JAMA.* 2022;328(10):921. https://doi.org/10.1001/jama.2022.14857
2. Nuzzo JB, Borio LL, Gostin LO. The WHO declaration of monkeypox as a global public health emergency. *JAMA.* 2022;328(7):615. https://doi.org/10.1001/jama.2022.12513
3. Daskalakis D, McClung RP, Mena L, et al. Monkeypox: avoiding the mistakes of past infectious disease epidemics. *Ann Intern Med.* 2022;175(8):1177–1178. https://doi.org/10.7326/M22-1748
4. Gonsalves GS, Mayer K, Beyrer C. Déjà vu all over again? Emergent monkeypox, delayed responses, and stigmatized populations. *J Urban Health.* 2022;99(4):603–606. https://doi.org/10.1007/s11524-022-00671-1
5. Goffman E. *Stigma: Notes on the Management of Spoiled Identity.* New York, NY: Simon & Schuster; 1963.
6. Hatzenbuehler ML, Phelan JC, Link BG. Stigma as a fundamental cause of population health inequalities. *Am J Public Health.* 2013;103(5):813–821. https://doi.org/10.2105/AJPH.2012.301069
7. Bayer R. Stigma and the ethics of public health: not can we but should we. *Soc Sci Med.* 2008;67(3):463–472. https://doi.org/10.1016/j.socscimed.2008.03.017
8. Volinn IJ. Health professionals as stigmatizers and destigmatizers of diseases: alcoholism and leprosy as examples. *Soc Sci Med.* 1983;17(7):385–393. https://doi.org/10.1016/0277-9536(83)90341-6
9. Hill B, Bergmeier H, Incollingo Rodriguez AC, et al. Weight stigma and obesity-related policies: a systematic review of the state of the literature. *Obes Rev.* 2021;22(11):e13333. https://doi.org/10.1111/obr.13333
10. Markel H. *Quarantine! East European Jewish Immigrants and the New York City Epidemics of 1892.* Baltimore, MD: Johns Hopkins University Press; 1999.
11. Poos LR. Lessons from past pandemics: disinformation, scapegoating, and social distancing. Available at: https://www.brookings.edu/blog/techtank/2020/03/16/lessons-from-past-pandemics-disinformation-scapegoating-and-social-distancing. Accessed November 1, 2022.
12. Pantelic M, Boyes M, Cluver L, Meinck F. HIV, violence, blame and shame: pathways of risk to internalized HIV stigma among South African adolescents living with HIV. *J Int AIDS Soc.* 2017;20(1):21771. https://doi.org/10.7448/IAS.20.1.21771
13. Tyler I. *Stigma: The Machinery of Inequality.* London, UK: Zed Books; 2021.
14. Hswen Y, Xu X, Hing A, Hawkins JB, Brownstein JS, Gee GC. Association of "#covid19" versus "#chinesevirus" with anti-Asian sentiments on Twitter: March 9–23, 2020. *Am J Public Health.* 2021;111(5):956–964. https://doi.org/10.2105/AJPH.2021.306154
15. Tran BX, Phan HT, Latkin CA, et al. Understanding global HIV stigma and discrimination: are contextual factors sufficiently studied? (GAP$_{RESEARCH}$). *Int J Environ Res Public Health.* 2019;16(11):1899. https://doi.org/10.3390/ijerph16111899
16. Mann J. Health and human rights: if not now, when? *Am J Public Health.* 2006;96(11):1940–1943. https://doi.org/10.2105/AJPH.96.11.1940
17. Monson S. Ebola as African: American media discourses of panic and otherization. *Afr Today.* 2017;63(3):3. https://doi.org/10.2979/africatoday.63.3.02
18. Wulfhorst E, Morgan DUS. CDC says returning Ebola medical workers should not be quarantined. October 27, 2014. Available at: https://www.reuters.com/article/us-health-ebola-usa-newyork-idUSKBN0IG12920141027. Accessed October 31, 2022.
19. Albertson B, Gadarian SK. *Anxious Politics: Democratic Citizenship in a Threatening World.* New York, NY: Cambridge University Press; 2015. https://doi.org/10.1017/CBO9781139963107
20. Ju W, Sannusi SN, Mohamad E. Stigmatizing monkeypox and COVID-19: a comparative framing study of the Washington Post's online news. *Int J Environ Res Public Health.* 2023;20(4):3347. https://doi.org/10.3390/ijerph20043347
21. Roh JS. Korea reports first confirmed monkeypox case, steps up monitoring. June 22, 2022. Available at: https://www.reuters.com/world/asia-pacific/skorea-reports-first-two-monkeypox-cases-yonhap-2022-06-21. Accessed February 24, 2023.
22. Choi J-h. Monkeypox feared to trigger fresh wave of homophobia. *Korea Herald.* July 7, 2022. Available at: https://www.koreaherald.com/view.php?ud=20220707000679. Accessed February 24, 2023.
23. Lee HJ. How much should Korea worry about monkeypox? *The Korea Times.* June 24, 2022. Available at: https://www.koreatimes.co.kr/www/nation/2023/02/119_331600.html. Accessed February 24, 2023.
24. Poushter J, Kent N. The global divide on homosexuality persists. June 25, 2020. Available at: https://www.pewresearch.org/global/2020/06/25/global-divide-on-homosexuality-persists. Accessed February 24, 2023.
25. Fisher M. A revealing map of the world's most and least ethnically diverse countries. *Washington Post.* May 16, 2013. Available at: https://www.washingtonpost.com/news/worldviews/wp/2013/05/16/a-revealing-map-of-the-worlds-most-and-least-ethnically-diverse-countries. Accessed February 18, 2023.
26. Boyon N. LGBT+ pride 2021 global survey—a 27-country Ipsos survey. Available at: https://www.ipsos.com/en/lgbt-pride-2021-global-survey-points-generation-gap-around-gender-identity-and-sexual-attraction. Accessed February 18, 2023.
27. Adida CL, Dionne KYR, Platas M. Ebola, elections, and immigration: how politicizing an epidemic can shape public attitudes. *Polit Groups Identities.* 2020;8(3):488–514. https://doi.org/10.1080/21565503.2018.1484376
28. Owens C, Hubach RD. Rural–urban differences in monkeypox behaviors and attitudes among men who have sex with men in the United States. *J Rural Health.* 2023;39(2):508–515. https://doi.org/10.1111/jrh.12726
29. Kim J, Bong Y, Lee JJ, Kang C. Over the rainbow: public attitude toward LGBT in South Korea. 2015. Available at: http://en.asaninst.org/contents/over-the-rainbow-public-attitude-toward-lgbt-in-south-korea. Accessed November 9, 2022.
30. Lee M, You M. Direct and indirect associations of media use with COVID-19 vaccine hesitancy in South Korea: cross-sectional Web-based survey. *J Med Internet Res.* 2022;24(1):e32329. https://doi.org/10.2196/32329
31. Lee M, Kang BA, You M. Knowledge, attitudes, and practices (KAP) toward COVID-19: a cross-sectional study in South Korea. *BMC Public Health.* 2021;21(1):295. https://doi.org/10.1186/s12889-021-10285-y
32. World Health Organization. Vaccines and immunization for monkeypox: interim guidance. November 16, 2022. Available at: https://www.who.int/publications/i/item/WHO-MPX-Immunization. Accessed June 25, 2023.
33. Daftary A, Frick M, Venkatesan N, Pai M. Fighting TB stigma: we need to apply lessons learnt from HIV activism. *BMJ Glob Health.* 2017;2(4):e000515. https://doi.org/10.1136/bmjgh-2017-000515
34. Kupferschmidt K. Why the monkeypox outbreak is mostly affecting men who have sex with men. *Science.* 2022;376(6600):1364–1365. https://doi.org/10.1126/science.add5966
35. Damaso CR. Phasing out monkeypox: mpox is the new name for an old disease. *Lancet Reg Health Am.* 2023;17:100424. https://doi.org/10.1016/j.lana.2022.100424

Erratum In: "Erratum In: 'Living Alone and Suicide Risk in the United States, 2008–2019'"

In: Erratum in: "Living Alone and Suicide Risk in the United States, 2008–2019." *Am J Public Health*. 2023;113(5):585.

When originally published, the online version of the erratum was posted online under an incorrect DOI. The DOI is: 10.2105/AJPH.2022.307080e. AJPH

https://doi.org/10.2105/AJPH.2023.307398

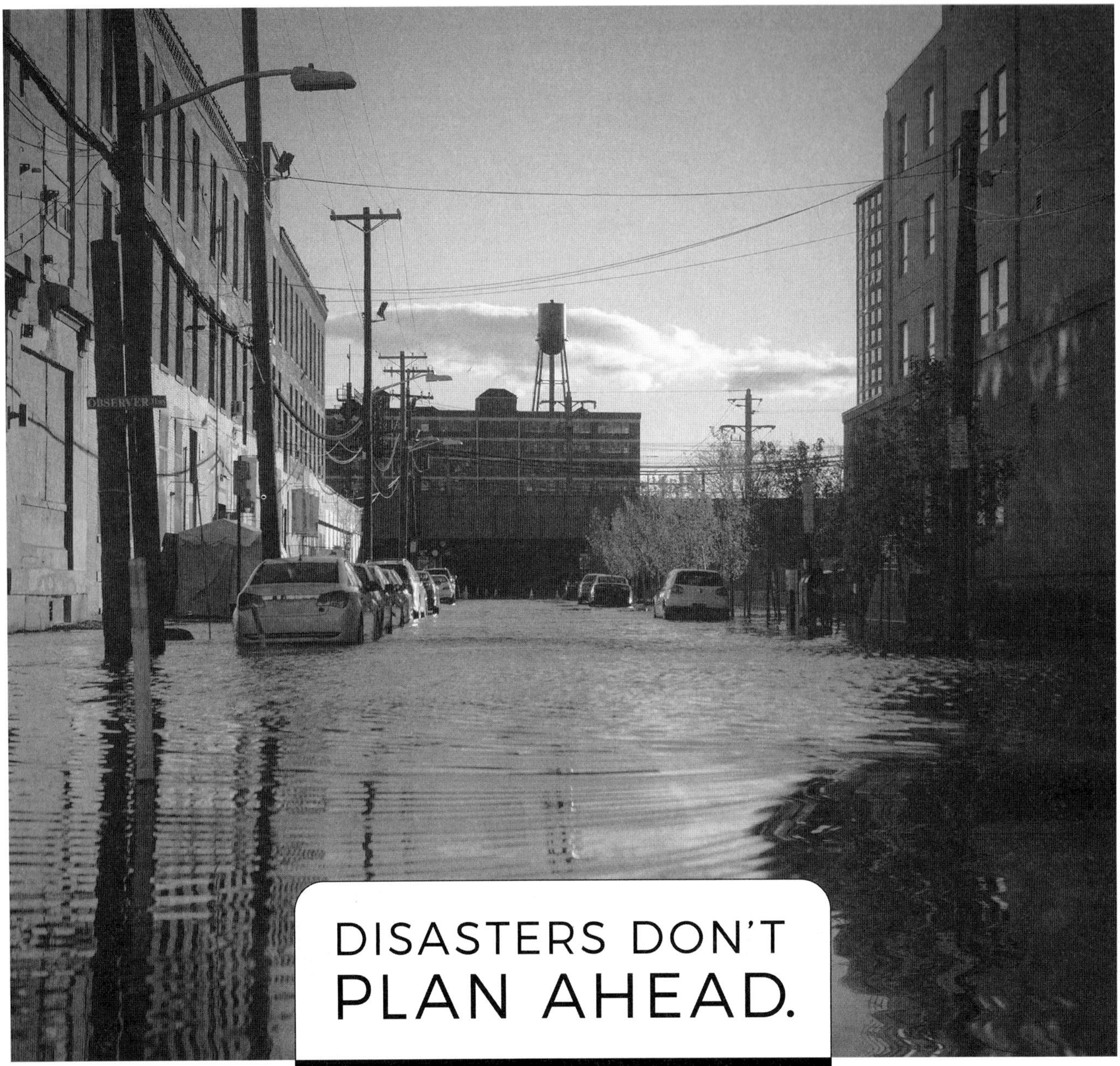

GET DOWN
WITH YOUR BLOOD PRESSURE™

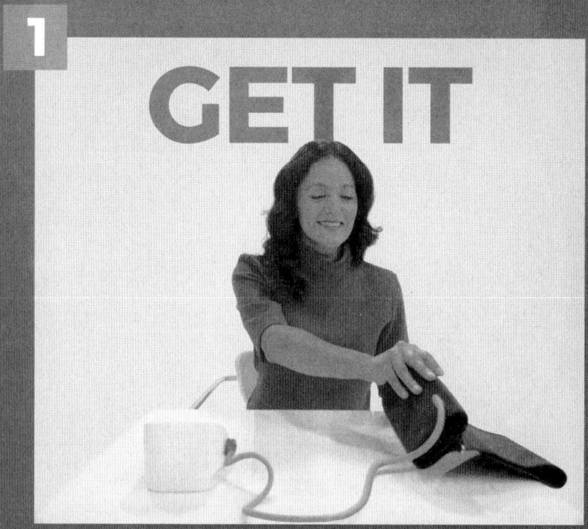

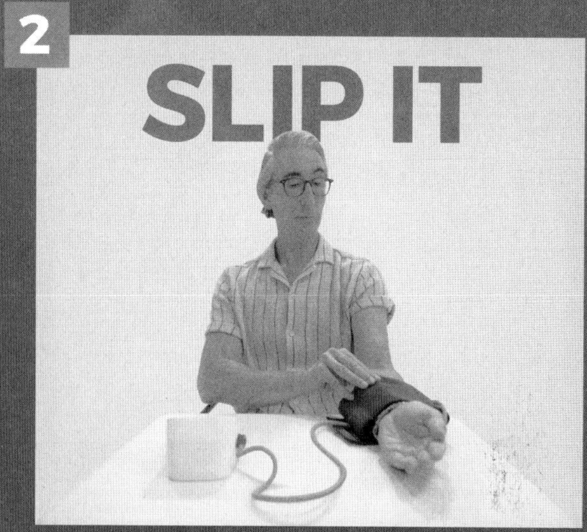

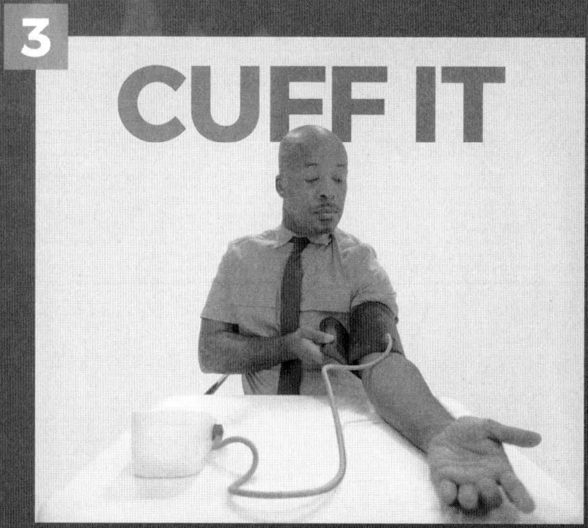

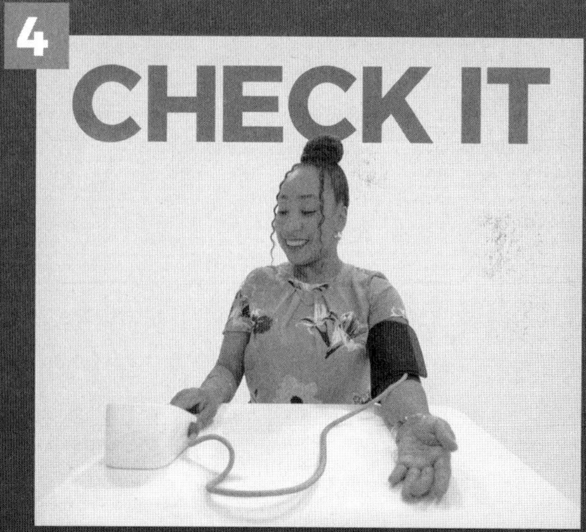

Check it every day. Self-monitoring is power.

ad COUNCIL

American Heart Association.

AMA AMERICAN MEDICAL ASSOCIATION

Visit: ManageYourBP.org

Or scan code for more.

In partnership with HHS Office of Minority Health and Health Resources and Services Administration under cooperative agreements CPIMP211227 and CPIMP211228.

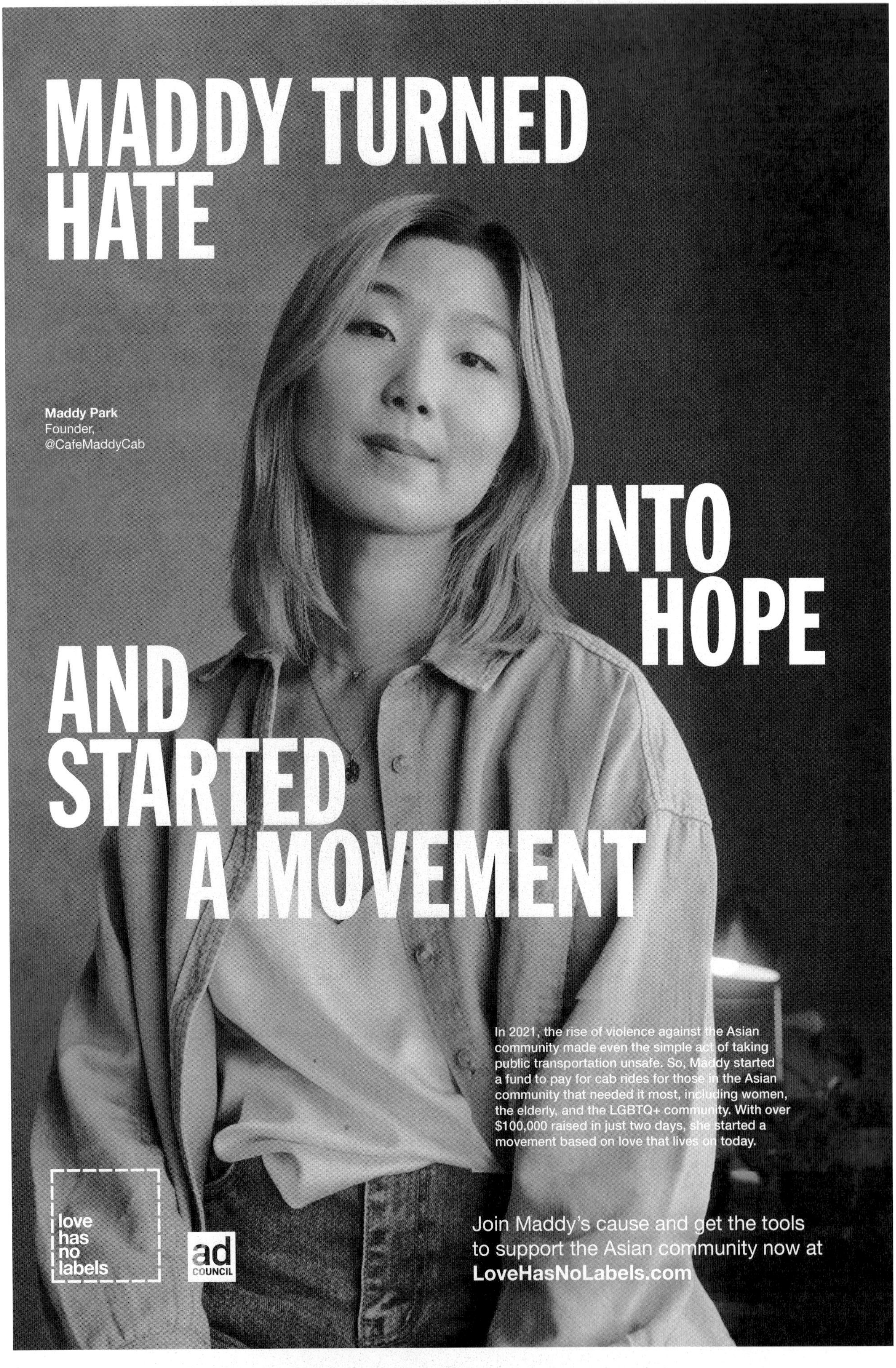
MADDY TURNED HATE
INTO HOPE
AND STARTED A MOVEMENT
Maddy Park
Founder,
@CafeMaddyCab
In 2021, the rise of violence against the Asian community made even the simple act of taking public transportation unsafe. So, Maddy started a fund to pay for cab rides for those in the Asian community that needed it most, including women, the elderly, and the LGBTQ+ community. With over $100,000 raised in just two days, she started a movement based on love that lives on today.
Join Maddy's cause and get the tools to support the Asian community now at
LoveHasNoLabels.com
love has no labels
ad COUNCIL

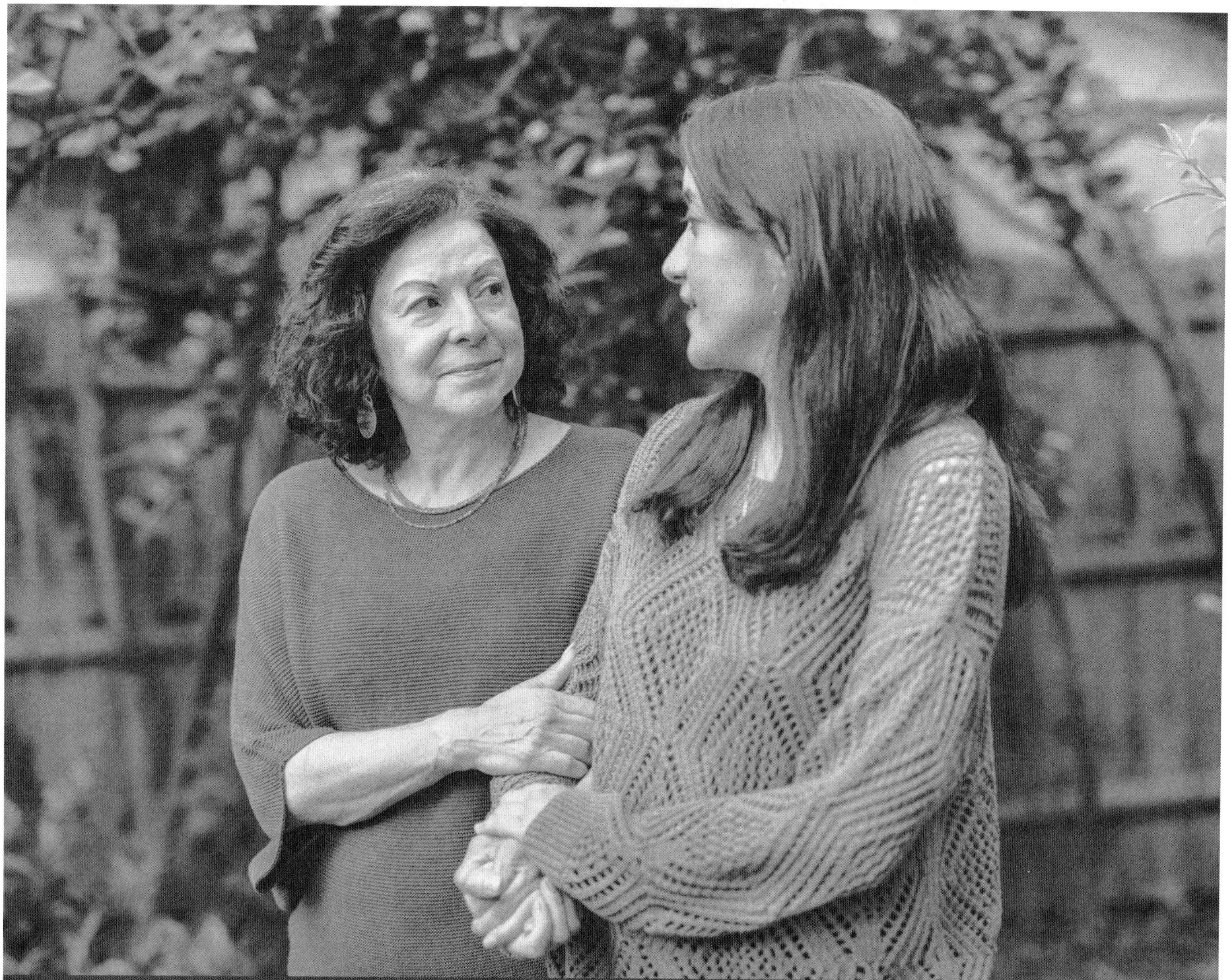

APHA 2023
ANNUAL MEETING & EXPO
ATLANTA | NOV. 12 – 15

UNABLE TO TRAVEL?

We're hosting a digital version of **APHA 2023 on Nov. 9-15**. This will include live virtual sessions on Thursday, Nov. 9 and access to all scientific session recordings from the in-person meeting. **You'll even be able to participate live in the Featured and General Sessions.**

CAN'T MISS SESSIONS

SATURDAY, NOV. 11
WOMEN'S LEADERSHIP INSTITUTE | 10 A.M. - 2:30 P.M.
Finding Your Impact and Influence

SUNDAY, NOV. 12
CHAMPION CONVERSATION | 2:30 – 4 P.M.
Public Health Emergency! U.S. Declining Health Status

CHAMPION CONVERSATION | 4:30 – 6 P.M.
America Dissected Podcast Live: Public Health & the Internet: Social Media, AI and the Future of Public Health
Host: Abdul El-Sayed, MD, DPhil

MONDAY, NOV. 13
GENERAL SESSION | 4:30 – 6 P.M.
We Dissent: Ensuring Equity In Public Health Education

TUESDAY, NOV. 14
CHAMPION CONVERSATION | 2:30 – 4 P.M.
The Economic Burden of Health Inequity:
A Social Justice Issue and Economic Imperative

WEDNESDAY, NOV. 15
CLOSING SESSION | 2:30 – 4 P.M.
Public Health Reimagined: Building a National System

Explore the full schedule, presenters and sessions at APHA.ORG/PROGRAM.

SUNDAY, NOV. 12
OPENING SESSION | 11 A.M. ET

KEYNOTE SPEAKER
Rachel L. Levine, MD
Admiral, U.S. Public Health Service
Assistant Secretary for Health
U.S. Department of Health and Human Services

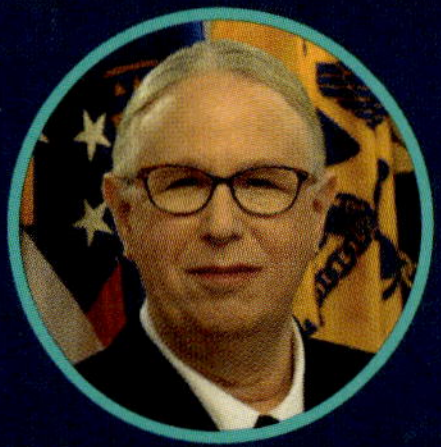

2023 FRIES PRIZE FOR IMPROVING HEALTH RECIPIENTS

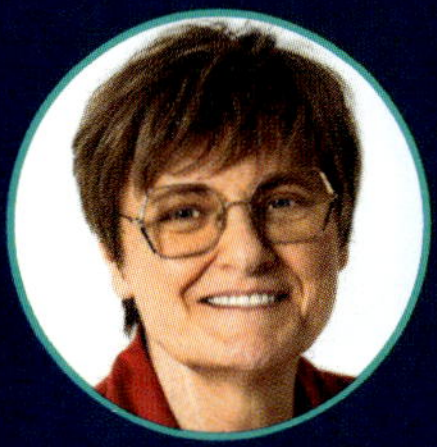

Katalin Karikó, PhD,
biochemist and researcher best known for her contributions to mRNA technology and the COVID-19 vaccines

Anne Schuchat, MD,
former principal deputy director,
Centers for Disease Control and Prevention

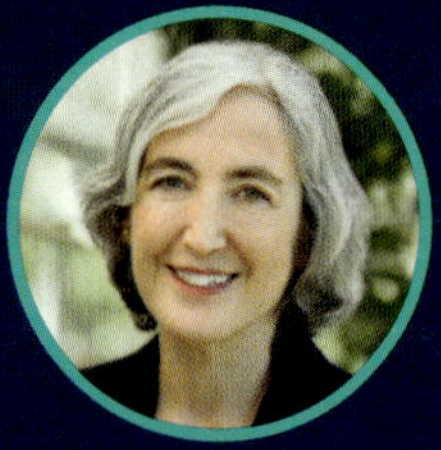

REGISTER AND RESERVE YOUR ROOM WITH AN OFFICIAL HOTEL TODAY!

APHA.org/AnnualMeeting